HEALTH CARE ISSUES, COSTS AND ACCESS

HEALTHCARE QUALITY IN THE U.S.

Health Care Issues, Costs and Access

Additional books in this series can be found on Nova's website under the Series tab.

Additional E-books in this series can be found on Nova's website under the E-book tab.

HEALTH CARE ISSUES, COSTS AND ACCESS

HEALTHCARE QUALITY IN THE U.S.

JOHN V. ELSWORTH
EDITOR

Nova Science Publishers, Inc.
New York

For permission to use material from this book please contact us:
Telephone 631-231-7269; Fax 631-231-8175
Web Site: http://www.novapublishers.com

LIBRARY OF CONGRESS CATALOGING-IN-PUBLICATION DATA

Healthcare quality in the U.S. / editor, John V. Elsworth.
p. ; cm.
Includes bibliographical references and index.
ISBN 978-1-61761-467-5 (hardcover)
1. Medical care--United States. 2. Medical care--United States--Quality control. I. Elsworth, John V.
[DNLM: 1. Quality of Health Care--United States. W 84.4 AA1]
RA395.A3H4136 2010
362.10973--dc22

2010034010

Published by Nova Science Publishers, Inc. † New York

CONTENTS

PREFACE

Health care seeks to diagnose, treat, and improve the physical and mental well-being of all Americans. Across the lifespan, health care helps people stay healthy, recover from illness, live with chronic disease or disability, and cope with death and dying. Quality health care delivers these services in a way that is safe, timely, patient centered, efficient, and equitable. Unfortunately, Americans too often do not receive care that they need, or they receive care that causes harm. This book examines the status of health care quality in the United States, targets where improvement is most needed, and explores how the quality of health care delivered to Americans is changing over time

Chapter 1- Problems with quality of health care in the United States earned the attention of the public with, and have steadily gained in importance since, the release of the first in a series of Institute of Medicine (IOM) reports on this topic, "To Err is Human: Building A Safer Health System," in 1999. The release of the IOM report represented a changing approach to addressing suboptimal health care quality, from one focused primarily on quality assurance to one focused on quality improvement broadly through the realignment of systems of delivering and financing care to incentivize quality of care. This issue now occupies a prominent position on the national agenda for health care reform and is the subject of considerable congressional interest.

Policy makers and others have offered a wide range of policy options to improve health care quality. This chapter provides information on the issue of quality measurement, which serves as the basis of several of the options policy makers are offering for addressing this problem. Specifically, recently introduced health reform bills have included a strong focus on supporting and expanding a coordinated national quality-measurement infrastructure. These include efforts that would broadly support the development of national priorities in the area of performance measurement; the development of new quality measures and identification of gaps in existing measures; the expansion of the endorsement process for quality measures; and the delineation of a process, in rulemaking, for selecting and implementing new quality measures for use in public health care programs.

Chapter 2- Health care seeks to diagnose, treat, and improve the physical and mental well-being of all Americans. Across the lifespan, health care helps people stay healthy, recover from illness, live with chronic disease or disability, and cope with death and dying. Quality health care delivers these services in a way that is safe, timely, patient centered, efficient, and equitable.[1] Unfortunately, Americans too often do not receive care that they need, or they receive care that causes harm. Care can also be delivered too late or without full consideration of a patient's preferences and values. Many times, our system of health care distributes services inefficiently and unevenly across populations.

Each year since 2003, the Agency for Healthcare Research and Quality (AHRQ), together with its partners in the Department of Health and Human Services (HHS), has reported on progress and opportunities for improving health care quality, as mandated by the U.S. Congress. The information amassed for the National Healthcare Quality Report (NHQR) since its inception is a growing knowledge base that can be used to address three critically important questions:

In: Healthcare Quality in the U.S.
Editor: John V. Elsworth
ISBN: 978-1-61761-467-5

Chapter 1

MEASURING HEALTH CARE QUALITY: MEASURE DEVELOPMENT, ENDORSEMENT, AND IMPLEMENTATION

Amanda K. Sarata

SUMMARY

Problems with quality of health care in the United States earned the attention of the public with, and have steadily gained in importance since, the release of the first in a series of Institute of Medicine (IOM) reports on this topic, "To Err is Human: Building A Safer Health System," in 1999. The release of the IOM report represented a changing approach to addressing suboptimal health care quality, from one focused primarily on quality assurance to one focused on quality improvement broadly through the realignment of systems of delivering and financing care to incentivize quality of care. This issue now occupies a prominent position on the national agenda for health care reform and is the subject of considerable congressional interest.

Policy makers and others have offered a wide range of policy options to improve health care quality. This chapter provides information on the issue of quality measurement, which serves as the basis of several of the options policy makers are offering for addressing this problem. Specifically, recently introduced health reform bills have included a strong focus on supporting and expanding a coordinated national quality-measurement infrastructure. These include efforts that would broadly support the development of national priorities in the area of performance measurement; the development of new quality measures and identification of gaps in existing measures; the expansion of the endorsement process for quality measures; and the delineation of a process, in rulemaking, for selecting and implementing new quality measures for use in public health care programs.

This chapter begins with a brief description of health care quality activity conceptually, the types of quality information that support these activities, and how quality measurement can be placed within these frameworks. It provides a discussion of the definition of quality measurement and a description of the life cycle of quality measures, including the development of quality measures (across provider types), the process of endorsement of quality measures, and the process for implementing those measures. Overviews of selected examples of implementation, including the Physician Quality Reporting Initiative (PQRI) and the Reporting Hospital Quality Data for Annual Payment Update (RHQDAPU), are included. The report concludes with an overview of key technical and policy issues in quality measurement.

Problems with quality of health care in the United States earned the attention of the public with, and have steadily gained in importance since, the release of the first in a series of Institute of Medicine (IOM) reports on this topic, "To Err is Human: Building A Safer Health System," in 1999. The release of the IOM report represented a changing approach to addressing suboptimal health care quality, from one focused primarily on quality assurance to one focused on quality improvement broadly through the realignment of systems of delivering and financing care to incentivize quality of care. This issue now occupies a prominent position on the national agenda for health care reform and is the subject of considerable congressional interest.

Policy makers and others have offered a wide range of policy options to improve health care quality. This chapter provides information on the issue of quality measurement, which serves as the basis of several of the options policy makers are offering for addressing this problem. Specifically, recently introduced health reform bills have included a strong focus on supporting and expanding a coordinated national quality measurement infrastructure. These include efforts that would broadly support the development of national priorities in the area of performance measurement; the development of new quality measures and identification of gaps in existing measures; the expansion of the endorsement process for quality measures; and the delineation of a process, in rulemaking, for selecting and implementing new quality measures for use in public health care programs.

This chapter begins with a brief description of health care quality activity conceptually, the types of quality information that support these activities, and how quality measurement can be placed within these frameworks. It provides a discussion of the definition of quality measurement and a description of the life cycle of quality measures, including the development of quality measures (across provider types); the process of endorsement of quality measures; and the process for implementing those measures. Overviews of selected examples of implementation, including the Physician Quality Reporting Initiative (PQRI) and the Reporting Hospital Quality Data for Annual Payment Update (RHQDAPU), are included. The report concludes with an overview of key technical and policy issues in quality measurement.

THE HEALTH CARE QUALITY PROBLEM

The U.S. health care system is characterized by systemic quality shortcomings. The IOM stated in 2001 that "[c]rucial reports from disciplined review bodies document the scale and gravity of the problems. Quality problems are everywhere, affecting many patients. Between the health care we have and the care we could have lies not just a gap, but a chasm."[1]

Significant activity has been undertaken to improve the quality of care delivered in the United States over the past decade, but a number of concerning trends remain.

The U.S health care system's quality problems are evidenced by a broad range of relevant quality indicators. These include high rates of medical and medication error; a high amenable mortality rate; overuse, underuse, and misuse of health care services; and a lack of, and variation in, diffusion of evidence-based guidelines.

In its 1999 study, the IOM reported that between 44,000 and 98,000 people die each year because of preventable medical errors, at a cost of between $17 billion and $29 billion per year. Serious adverse medication events are estimated to occur in up to 15% of hospitalized patients, and more than 100,000 deaths are attributed annually to such reactions.[2] A July 2008 study reports that despite spending two times more per capita than any other major industrialized country on health care, the United States has an amenable mortality rate—deaths that are amenable to health care intervention and may have been prevented by that intervention—of 110 per 100,000 (ranking 19th out of 19 surveyed countries).[3]

With respect to the problems of overuse, misuse, and underuse of health care services, a study conducted by the Midwest Business Group on Health in 2003 found that approximately "30 percent of all direct health care outlays are the result of poor-quality care, consisting primarily of overuse, misuse and waste."[4] Another study found that as many as 20% to 30% of patients received contraindicated care.[5] In addition, a 2007 RAND study found that only 46.5% of children receive care recommended by evidence-based guidelines, and a similar RAND study conducted in 2003 concluded that adults receive only 55% of indicated care.[6]

According to the IOM, an average of 17 years is required for findings from randomized clinical trials to be implemented into clinical practice, and when they are, it is done so in an uneven fashion.[7] Taken together, these findings evidence significant shortfalls in the quality of care provided in the United States.

Conceptualizing Health Care Quality

Despite the fact that most experts agree that health care quality is a serious problem deserving of attention, a precise operational definition for the concept can be difficult to identify. Although there is no single universally agreed upon definition for quality of care, or health care quality, perhaps the most commonly cited definition is the IOM's definition, as follows: "(t)he degree to which health services for individuals and populations increase the likelihood of desired health outcomes and are consistent with current professional knowledge."[8]

The 2001 IOM report "Crossing the Quality Chasm" further defines quality of care in terms of six domains:

- *Effective.* Providing services based on scientific knowledge to all who could benefit.
- *Efficient.* Avoiding waste, including waste of equipment, supplies, ideas, and energy.
- *Equitable.* Providing care that does not vary in quality because of personal characteristics.
- *Patient-centered.* Providing care that is responsive to and respectful of individual patient preferences.

- *Safe*. Avoiding injuries to patients from the care that is supposed to help them.
- *Timely*. Reducing waits and sometimes-harmful delays.

Most health care quality efforts aim to improve one or more of these six domains of quality of care, and quality care is often colloquially defined as simply delivering the right care to the right person at the right time. However basic it may appear, operationalizing these six domains, and thus improving health care quality, has proven difficult.

The effort to improve health care quality is operationally embodied by a wide range of quality activities. One way to consider these activities is by grouping them into one or more of the following four areas: (1) research (basic, translational, and health services); (2) quality measurement; (3) quality reporting (encompassing both increased transparency and incentive alignment); and (4) patient safety activities.[9] Reliable and sound quality information plays a fundamental role in all of these health care quality activities, which may both use and generate such information. For those activities that rely on quality information, such as quality reporting, their effectiveness is directly dependent upon the quality of the information available. There are various types of quality information, including evidence syntheses, health technology assessments, clinical comparative effectiveness data, clinical practice guidelines, quality measure data, and medical error/near miss reports. In many cases, these different types of information are interrelated. For example, evidence syntheses are utilized as the basis for the development of clinical practice guidelines, which in many cases in turn serve as the basis for developing quality measures.

Quality information may be broadly leveraged through the types of activities referenced above for a number of purposes, including to educate and inform providers about performance; for public reporting to inform consumer decision making; to create payment incentives; to inform accreditation or maintenance of certification; to inform internal quality assurance or improvement efforts; for public health surveillance efforts and activities; and to inform system-level changes to improve safety. Quality information may be fed back to inform the modification of quality measures, incentive programs, quality assurance activities, health care provider education, or the processes of delivering health care with the goal of improving quality.

This chapter focuses specifically on quality measurement, one subset of quality activities, and will focus on the processes used to develop, endorse, select, and implement quality measures.

Overview of Quality Measurement

Broadly, quality measurement focuses on assessing processes, structures, and outcomes of health care, and for this reason, quality measures are informally categorized as structural, process, or outcome measures. This model of quality measurement rests on the premise that a sound structure will support appropriate processes of care that in turn will result in good outcomes.[10] Ideally, process measures are supported by research demonstrating a link to improved outcomes, and all measures will assess things that are under the direct control of the health care system.

Structural measures assess whether "the resources and organizational arrangements are in place to deliver care," for example, staffing ratios or health information technology (HIT) implementation. Process measures assess whether the "appropriate provider activities are carried out to deliver care," for example, percentage of indicated patients receiving mammograms within a given timeframe. Finally, outcomes measures assess "the results of physician and other provider activities," for example, 30-day mortality rates post-hospitalization for pneumonia.[11] Composite measures, which summarize performance across separate and discrete measures of quality, are a useful tool for certain end-users, such as policy makers and the general public. [12] The Centers for Medicare and Medicaid Services (CMS) now includes several Agency for Healthcare Research and Quality (AHRQ)-developed composite measures in its Reporting Hospital Quality Data for Annual Payment Update (RHQDAPU) program (described later in this chapter).

In addition, quality measures may be developed in order to collect patients' reports of system performance. An example of this type of measure may be found in the Consumer Assessment of Healthcare Providers and Systems (CAHPS) survey and the Hospital Consumer Assessment of Healthcare Providers and Systems (HCAHPS) survey, both funded by AHRQ. While these measures may assess the delivery of evidence- or consensus-based clinical care, they also include an evaluation of the human aspects of how that care was delivered.

Quality measures may attempt to assess or evaluate one of three broader breakdowns in health care quality: (1) overuse of health care services, (2) misuse of health care services, or (3) underuse of health care services. This approach encompasses variation in care patterns as well as disparities in quality of care received. The development of quality measures may be based either on existing clinical practice guidelines (evidence-based) or on consensus-based guidelines. Generally, utilizing an evidence-based guideline as a basis for a quality measure is preferred over using a consensus-based one; however, as there are significant gaps in the evidence base, in many cases, consensus-based guidelines are the only option available. Although the development of reliable and valid quality measures tends to be challenging, the development of structural and process quality measures may be less complicated than the development and specification of outcomes measures, which requires complex risk-adjustment manipulations to account for variation in patient case-mix. Data sources for quality measures vary, but include four primary sources: (1) administrative claims data, (2) medical records, (3) medical registries, and (4) patients' reports.

Quality measures may be used for a number of purposes. They may be used to assess performance at the level of a hospital (or other health care facility, for example, a nursing home or outpatient surgical center); a health care provider, group of providers, or practice group; or a health plan. They may be used by payers, purchasers, health care consumers, regulators, accrediting or licensure bodies, researchers, health care providers, or health care facilities. Finally, quality measures may be used as the basis for policies that realign payment incentives; to facilitate internal quality improvement or quality assurance efforts; to empower consumer decision making; or to provide feedback on performance—for the purposes of self-improvement— to health care providers, health plans, or health care facilities.

The life cycle of a quality measure is composed of three basic components: the creation and specification of the measure, the endorsement of the measure, and the selection and implementation of the measure. This process may not always be perfectly linear in all cases (for example, an entity may adapt an existing endorsed measure for use in one of its quality-related activities), but with respect to the creation of *de novo* quality measures, these are the ordered steps generally followed. Each stage is discussed in more detail in the following sections.

DEFINITION OF OVERUSE, MISUSE, AND UNDERUSE OF HEALTH CARE SERVICES

Overuse occurs when a service is provided even though its risk of harm exceeds its likely benefit— that is, when it is not warranted on medical grounds.

Misuse includes incorrect diagnoses as well as medical errors and other sources of avoidable complications.

Underuse occurs when a service that would have been medically beneficial is not provided.

Source: Adapted from Congressional Budget Office. "The Overuse, Underuse and Misuse of Health Care." Testimony before the Committee on Finance, U.S. Senate. July 17, 2008.

There is a wide range of current efforts to develop quality metrics that may be used in performance measurement activities and, likewise, there are a number of different entities involved in the development, endorsement, selection, and implementation of quality measures. AHRQ reports in its 2008 National Healthcare Quality Report that the "often opportunistic, incremental, and fragmented development of quality measures without detailed consideration of data sources, analysis and maintenance requirements, and user needs" is a challenge, and that "uncoordinated and isolated measure development can lead different groups to create and advocate competing and sometimes conflicting measures of the same process or outcome."[13]

In an attempt to better coordinate performance measurement and other quality activities, in November of 2008, the National Quality Forum (NQF) convened the National Priorities Partnership (NPP), a collaborative effort between 28 key health care stakeholders representing all major health care perspectives.[14] The goal of the NPP is to rapidly improve quality in six priority areas, including patient and family engagement, population health, safety, care coordination, overuse, and palliative and end-of-life care. The NPP aims to achieve measurable progress in these six areas, specifically focusing on payment, public reporting, quality improvement, and consumer engagement.

The Medicare Improvements for Patients and Providers Act of 2008 (MIPPA, P.L. 110-275) further emphasized the importance of "an integrated national strategy and priorities for health care performance measurement in all applicable settings."[15] MIPPA required the Secretary to enter into a contract with a consensus-based entity (and provided as an example the National Quality Forum) to help strengthen and better focus the nation's performance-measurement infrastructure, and specifically to synthesize evidence and convene stakeholders to provide recommendations on a national performance-measurement infrastructure; to endorse and maintain measures; and to report annually to the Secretary on these activities. The National Quality Forum was awarded this contract and recently released its first report, *Improving Healthcare Performance: Setting Priorities and Enhancing Measurement Capacity*, in fulfillment of this statutory requirement. [16]

Development of Quality Measures

The initial phase in the life cycle of a quality measure is the development stage. In this stage, measures are conceived of, created, specified, refined, and oftentimes field tested. Quality measures are developed by a number of different measure developers, including The Joint Commission, the National Committee for Quality Assurance (NCQA), and the American Medical Association (AMA)-convened Physician Consortium for Performance Improvement (PCPI), for application in a wide variety of settings, including hospitals, nursing homes, clinics, and to evaluate health plans.

Measures may generally be developed in one of two ways: they may be created entirely anew, or *de novo*, or existing measures may be identified and adapted for a specific purpose (i.e., hospital accreditation). Traditionally, developers have focused on measures of process rather than outcomes, and they generally direct their efforts toward developing measures focused on a specific setting (e.g., hospital) or in a particular clinical area (e.g., pneumonia). Gaps have occurred in measure development where services span provider settings or where no single entity has sole responsibility for providing a service (e.g., coordination of care or end-of-life care). In addition, measure development may be guided by overuse or cost intensiveness, or rather, may be guided by explicit links to improved outcomes, regardless of cost or cost burden. From a value- based purchasing perspective, development would ideally be guided by both; however, from the consumer perspective, outcomes may be more important than costs.

This section details the processes used by measure developers to develop quality measures for evaluating the performance of hospitals, physicians, and health plans. An examination of these processes reveals that they share several attributes: they all solicit public input on measures, they all rely on panels or workgroups of technical and/or clinical specialists for guidance, and they all subject measures to some degree of field testing. In addition, both the Joint Commission and NCQA utilize a set of clearly delineated and specific attributes by which to assess and evaluate measures' value and thus guide their development activities. NQF has recognized the importance of testing quality measures by instituting a mechanism of "time-limited" endorsement for a period of 12-24 months for those measures that meet all of NQF 's standards for endorsement, but that have not been subjected to rigorous field testing.[17]

Hospital Measures

The Joint Commission has one of the most well-developed and clearly specified processes of quality-measure development, and has been involved in developing performance measures since 1986 for hospitals (these measures may be used by other health care organizations, including home care, behavioral health care and long term care organizations). Reporting quality data was made a formal requirement for Joint Commission hospital accreditation in 1998.

The Joint Commission, formerly the Joint Commission on the Accreditation of Healthcare Organizations, or JCAHO, is a private, non-profit organization that establishes quality and safety standards and accredits health care organizations for participation in federal health insurance programs. For example, The Joint Commission accredits approximately 80% of hospitals for participation in Medicare by assessing their compliance with standards related to patient rights and education, infection control, preventing medical errors, medical staffing ratios, and data- collection processes. The organization describes its mission as "continuously improving the safety and quality of care provided to the public through the provision of health care accreditation and related services that support performance improvement in health care organizations."[18]

When The Joint Commission began its work in the area of quality measurement in 1986, it focused on developing quality measures completely *de novo*, an involved and resource-intensive endeavor. However, while The Joint Commission was engaged in this work, many other measure developers began developing and implementing their own measures. For this reason, The Joint Commission changed course in the mid-1990s and redirected its efforts toward adapting (evaluating and testing) existing quality measures for its purposes. This shift resulted in the creation of a standardized process for adapting existing measures consisting of a series of specific steps. The Joint Commission focuses on developing its measures in sets, and defines a "core measure set" as "a unique grouping of performance measures, carefully selected to provide, when viewed together, a robust picture of the care provided in a given focus area."[19]

Initial measure develcpment requires significant preliminary work, including a review of the literature to evaluate the evidence base and identify existing measures in a particular topical area. The findings from this review are summarized and serve as the basis of a measurement framework, which is used throughout the development process. The first formal step in the process is the empanelling of a group of experts with balance as a key focus. This expert advisory panel includes representation from relevant medical, nursing, and pharmacy professionals, as well as state hospital associations, consumers, and CMS. Funders are not represented on these panels to avoid conflicts of interest, and full disclosure is required of all members.

After the panel has been convened, The Joint Commission issues a "call for measures" to solicit measures from all known measure developers. The measures received are vetted by staff, and evaluated against The Joint Commission's attributes of core performance measures and associated evaluation criteria. These criteria include the following:

- Measures target improvement in the health of populations.
- Measures are precisely defined and specified.
- Measures are reliable.
- Measures are valid.
- Measures are easily interpreted by users.
- Measures are risk-adjusted or stratified.
- Measures are under provider control.
- Measures have publicly available measure constructs.
- Measures are useful in the accreditation process.
- Measures rely on accessible data and low-cost data collection efforts.

There is significant overlap between The Joint Commission's measure attributes, NQF's measure evaluation criteria, and NCQA's desirable measure attributes.[20]

Measures that meet these criteria are forwarded to the expert advisory panel, and final candidate measures are posted to The Joint Commission's website, where they undergo a 30-day comment period. Measures are adjusted according to the feedback received during the comment period, at which point general specifications may be formulated and field testing begun. The Joint Commission's field testing is well developed, and involves both alpha testing—for feasibility and utility—and beta testing—for reliability, validity, and cost, among other things. There are opportunities for measure adjustment and refinement at all points in this process. Based on the results of the field testing, the expert advisory panel recommends implementation of a set of final measures, and the measures will then be integrated into ORYX, the performance measurement component of The Joint Commission's accreditation process.

Physician Measures

The American Medical Association (AMA)-convened Physician Consortium for Performance Improvement (PCPI) is a physician-led, multi-stakeholder group that has taken the lead in the development of quality measures for physicians. The Consortium, staffed by the AMA and led by a 23-member Executive Board, is composed of more than 100 national and state medical societies, experts in methodology and data collection, AHRQ, and CMS. The PCPI supports, and provides in-kind resources for, the establishment of topic-specific work groups that include both clinician specialists as well as technical methodological experts to develop disease- or condition specific-measures.

To date, the PCPI has developed more than 250 measures in over 40 clinical areas, and the measures are heavily used by CMS's Physician Quality Reporting Initiative (PQRI). In addition, uses for these measures include integration into electronic health records (EHRs), Maintenance of Certification (MOC) for physicians, and CMS demonstration projects, and measures may be used for quality improvement purposes, as well as for accountability.

The process used by PCPI to develop measures is not as longstanding as are those employed by The Joint Commission and NCQA, simply by virtue of the fact that the organization is far younger. While The Joint Commission began developing hospital performance measures in 1986, and NCQA began developing its HEDIS measures in 1992, the PCPI was established in 2000 to help guide medical specialty groups in generating physician-level measures, at least partially in anticipation of a formal, statutorily established physician quality reporting system for Medicare- participating physicians. The scope and depth of PCPI's work was described in late 2007 as nascent;[21] however, PCPI has had the advantage of being able to draw on existing work in this area, and quickly developed its own robust process for measure development (see Figure A-2).

PCPI has been endeavoring to make strategic changes in emphasis as it matures. It has refocused its measure-development efforts, and requires the following three criteria be met by any topic prior to proceeding with development in the area:

1. The topic is an area designated as high impact (by the IOM, NPP, etc.).
2. The topic is a gap area or an area with high variation in care.
3. The topic has an adequate evidence base.

If these three criteria are met, PCPI evaluates whether the topic under consideration is likely to generate measures in the following four areas, which it terms "high value": care coordination, patient safety, appropriateness/overuse, and quality improvement collaboratives. The Consortium has also shifted its focus to developing a comprehensive "core" measure set.

After a topic has been approved, an topic-specific expert work group is convened, consisting of two co-chairs with expertise in the clinical area as well as in measure-development methodology; clinicians in all relevant areas; methodologists; guideline experts; patients, purchasers, consumer groups and health plans; and sometimes coding experts, depending on the topical area. Importantly, representatives from The Joint Commission and NCQA are included in the composition of the work groups to ensure measure harmonization to the greatest extent possible.

Prior to beginning its actual measure drafting, the work group conducts a literature review (and review of the existing evidence base) and identifies desired outcomes (with respect to either a certain condition or procedure). The work group meets once in person and conducts several conference calls to facilitate the measure-drafting process, after which public comment is solicited on the measures. The work group will then review the comments and incorporate them as necessary. The revised measures are then submitted for approval to PCPI. Measure testing is undertaken on the measures to assess both reliability and feasibility, and then measures are submitted to NQF for potential endorsement and also released for public use.

Plan Measures

The National Committee for Quality Assurance (NCQA), a private, 501(c)(3) not-for-profit organization dedicated to improving health care quality through the accreditation of health plans and quality-measure development, has taken the lead role in the development of quality measures used to evaluate health plans. Its programs, which focus on evaluating the performance of health plans, also include the development of report cards, public-policy documents, and educational activities.

Perhaps NCQA's most well-known performance evaluation tool is the Healthcare Effectiveness Data and Information Set (HEDIS), a set of standardized measures used by more than 90% of health plans to measure clinical performance in areas such as medication use, control of high blood pressure, breast cancer screening, immunization, and comprehensive diabetes care, among others. HEDIS 2009 consists of quality measures in eight health care domains, and may be used to assess clinical quality in both managed care organizations (MCOs) and preferred-provider organizations (PPOs).

HEDIS measures are developed by NCQA using a process involving input from a broad range of stakeholders, including purchasers, policy makers, health care providers, patients, and health plans (see Figure A-3). There are several key groups involved in this process: Technical Advisory Groups (TAGs) provide guidance on methodological considerations; the Committee on Performance Measurement (CPM) provides guidance throughout the measure-development process and makes final decisions regarding adoption; and Measurement

Advisory Panels (MAPs) report to the CPM and provide specialized guidance for measure development in a specific area.

The process begins with the identification of a topic, a literature review, and measure identification. Measures are evaluated for inclusion in the development process against a series of three key criteria: relevance, scientific soundness, and feasibility. A MAP is created to guide development, and initial measure specifications are drafted by the TAG and then presented to the MAP. Measures are then field tested, revisions are made, and then the measures are presented to the CPM. The revised measures are posted on the NCQA website for a period of 30 days, with a request for public comment. Finally, the CPM reviews all comments, revises the measures as needed based on the comments, and then votes formally to adopt the measures for inclusion in HEDIS.

The Role of the Centers for Medicare and Medicaid Services (CMS)

The Centers for Medicare and Medicaid Services (CMS) plays an important role in providing overall guidance for the development of measures for use in its multiple quality activities. This is reflected in an agency document entitled *Quality Measures Development Overview*, which explains that "CMS has developed a standardized approach for the development and maintenance of quality measures it uses in its various quality initiatives and programs."[22] This process, referred to by CMS as the Measures Management System and described in more detail below, involves participation by three main entities: CMS, a measure developer (e.g., PCPI or NCQA), and a Technical Expert Panel (TEP) whose responsibility it is to provide expert guidance to both CMS and the measure developer (see Figure A-1).

The measure-development process CMS has outlined is followed by the CMS-funded measure developer and shares many similarities with those employed by The Joint Commission, NCQA, and the PCPI. It begins with the definition of a topic and the empanelling of a topic-specific TEP. With the guidance of the TEP, the measure developer develops a measure framework, identifies candidate measures, and provides these measures, accompanied by general information, to the TEP for review. After the TEP reviews the candidate measures list, it is submitted to CMS for review and approval, and public comment may be solicited. Measures approved by CMS at this stage move forward to the specification-development stage. Once specifications have been created for the measures, they are approved by CMS, the measures are tested for both reliability and feasibility, and public comment is solicited. Refinements may be made to the measures at this point, based on public feedback, and they will go through a final approval process and then be submitted for consensus endorsement (e.g., to the NQF).

Although CMS relies on both TEPs and measure developers in the process of developing the quality measures it will employ in its quality programs, the agency itself plays a critical role at many points during this process. This distinction is not clearly delineated by the agency. In its recently released *Roadmap for Quality Measurement in the Traditional Medicare Fee-for-Service Program*, CMS states that "(i)n general, CMS does not play a significant role in the development or endorsement of quality measures."[23] This statement, in the context of the *Quality Measures Overview Document*, may understate the role of CMS in this process.

While CMS does not carry out the technical process of specifying quality measures (this task falls to the measure contractor), it is a critical part of the process at many points. CMS helps to define the topic for which measures will be developed; provides approval of candidate measures for specification; determines whether public comment will be required in the early stages of measure development (pre-specification); approves measure specifications; determines whether measures with specifications will be submitted for consensus review prior to testing; and gives final approval of measures for use in its programs after completion of testing and formal public comment. The agency plays a guiding role in the process and appears to make the final decisions regarding measure advancement.

The Role of the Agency for Healthcare Research and Quality (AHRQ)

The Agency for Healthcare Research and Quality (AHRQ) plays an important role in the development of quality measures. The agency's authorizing language stipulates that it shall conduct and support research, evaluations, and training; support demonstration projects, research networks, and multidisciplinary centers; provide technical assistance; and disseminate information on health care and on systems for the delivery of such care. This activity specifically targets the following areas:

- the quality, effectiveness, efficiency, appropriateness and value of health care services;
- quality measurement and improvement;
- the outcomes, cost, cost-effectiveness, and use of health care services and access to such services;
- clinical practice, including primary care and practice-oriented research;
- health care technologies, facilities, and equipment;
- health care costs, productivity, organization, and market forces;
- health promotion and disease prevention, including clinical preventive services;
- health statistics, surveys, database development, and epidemiology; and
- medical liability."[24]

AHRQ carries out a number of measure-development activities, including development of the Consumer Assessment of Healthcare Providers and Systems (CAHPS) survey, the AHRQ Quality Indicators, and the National Healthcare Quality and National Healthcare Disparities reports. The measures developed under these various activities are used both to track and report on quality at the national level (the National Healthcare Quality and National Healthcare Disparities reports) and to monitor quality at the institution level (CAHPS and the Quality Indicators).

The AHRQ Quality Indicators is a family of measurement indicators, including indicators focusing on prevention, inpatient care, patient safety, and pediatric care, that make use of hospital inpatient administrative data. For 2009, CMS has incorporated some of AHRQ's Patient Safety Indicators (PSIs) and Inpatient Quality Indicators (IQIs) into its Reporting Hospital Quality Data for Annual Payment Update (RHQDAPU) program. In addition, a modified version of the CAHPS survey, the Hospital Consumer Assessment of Healthcare

Providers and Systems (HCAHPS) survey, is used by CMS in its RHQDAPU program. This information is also publicly reported on CMS's Hospital Compare website.

ENDORSEMENT OF QUALITY MEASURES

The National Quality Forum (NQF) is the entity in the United States with the lead responsibility for endorsing quality measures. Numerous measure developers, including NCQA, PCPI, and The Joint Commission, submit their measures to NQF for endorsement, and other entities, including CMS, the Hospital Quality Alliance (HQA), medical boards, and health care providers, often choose quality measures for their quality activities from among the list of NQF-endorsed measures. The endorsement process provides a mechanism for recognizing those measures that meet certain standards and allows interested parties to identify easily a set of valid and reliable measures. This is valuable, given the large number of extant quality metrics.[25]

Many entities rely on NQF-endorsed measures for use in their quality activities. For example, CMS's Physician Quality Reporting Initiative (PQRI) is statutorily required in 2008 and 2009 to use measures that have been "adopted or endorsed by a consensus organization (such as the National Quality Forum or AQA)"[26] and is required in 2010 and subsequent years to use "such measures selected by the Secretary from measures that have been endorsed by the entity with a contract with the Secretary under section 1890(a) of the Social Security Act."[27] Also, with respect to CMS's Reporting Hospital Quality Data for Annual Payment Update (RHQDAPU) program, the Secretary is required to "add other measures that reflect consensus among affected parties and, to the extent feasible and practicable, shall include measures set forth by one or more national consensus building entities."[28]

National Quality Forum (NQF)

The National Quality Forum (NQF), a public-private not-for-profit membership organization with more than 350 members, was established in 1999 with the mission of improving the quality of health care, specifically through setting national goals for improvement, through endorsing quality measures, and through education and outreach to facilitate the realization of the quality goals it has recommended. The President's Advisory Commission on Consumer Protection and Quality in the Health Care Industry (the Quality Commission) recommended the establishment of what would later come to be known as NQF in a March 1998 report entitled "Quality First: Better Health Care for All Americans." This chapter recommended "establishing two complementary entities, one public and one private, to provide ongoing national leadership in health care quality improvement. The Commission recommends the creation of a broadly represented, publicly administered—Advisory Council for Health Care Quality—and a privately administered—Forum for Health Care Quality Measurement and Reporting."

The NQF is a voluntary consensus standards-setting organization, as defined in law by the National Technology Transfer Advancement Act (NTTAA) and by the Office of Management and Budget (OMB) Circular A-119. According to OMB Circular A-1 19, the five attributes of a voluntary consensus standards-setting body are balance, openness, due process, consensus, and having an appeals process.[29] Currently, NQF is the only body that meets these formal criterion as a voluntary consensus standards-setting body for health quality measures. In addition, the NTTAA requires federal agencies to use voluntary consensus standards in their activities, unless doing so conflicts with existing law or is impractical.[30]

NQF 's most prominent and visible role has been in its capacity as a national-level quality measure endorser (it also endorses frameworks, reporting practices, and preferred practices), and it has to date endorsed more than 500 quality measures. Its decisions are highly respected and valued by all stakeholders; however, because the endorsement process is laborious and methodical, and tends to be lengthy, measure endorsement cannot keep pace with measure development. NQF has begun to emphasize the importance of harmonizing measures, and places value, for example, on setting neutrality and common conventions for measures related to a specific condition or targeted group.

NQF utilizes a rigorous and methodical process by which it reviews and judges quality measures for potential endorsement, known formally as the consensus development process (CDP) (see Figure B-1). This process comprises seven formal steps: (1) the formation of a steering committee, (2) a call for measures, (3) measure evaluation, (4) public and member comment, (5) member voting, (6) consensus standards approval committee review, and (7) appeals.[31] To begin the process, NQF puts out a public call for members for a steering committee. It is the job of the committee to guide the evaluation process and provide expert input and guidance. The next steps entail a call for measures, where measure developers (not necessarily NQF members) are asked to submit their measures for consideration for endorsement. Developers have a period of 30 days during which to submit their measures.

Once measures have been collected, the steering committee begins the evaluation process. Measures are evaluated against four criteria, including the following:

- whether the measure is linked to gains in quality and health outcomes,
- whether the measure is reliable and valid,
- whether the measure is usable (results are easy to understand and useful), and
- whether the measure is feasible (ease of access to required data).

A measure is initially evaluated against the first criterion—the relationship between a measure and quality and health outcomes—and if it is judged to pass this threshold, it will then be evaluated against the remaining three criteria. A measure may fail to gain endorsement, for example, if it is judged to assess a core competency, rather than high-quality care.

For measures that survive this evaluation process, there is a 30-day public comment period, after which the public's comments are reviewed by the steering committee and incorporated as appropriate. At this time, the revised measures are posted and NQF members have a 30-day period during which they are invited to vote either in favor of or in opposition to endorsement. The final endorsement recommendation is made by the Consensus Standards Approval Committee (CSAC) to the NQF Board of Directors, which affirms the CSAC's recommendation. Appeals may be made for a 30-day period following ratification of endorsement by the NQF Board of Directors.

The Role of AQA Adoption

The AQA Alliance, formerly known as the Ambulatory Care Quality Alliance, was established in 2004 and is co-sponsored by the Agency for Healthcare Research and Quality (AHRQ), the American College of Physicians (ACP), the American Academy of Family Physicians (AAFP), and America's Health Insurance Plans (AHIP). AQA is a consensus organization with broad stakeholder representation, which until recently "adopted" physician-quality measures, a status which served as AQA's recommendation that a measure is ready for implementation. During this process, AQA considered measures that were either NQF-endorsed, or would be going through the NQF-endorsement process, for adoption. If an AQA-adopted measure went through the NQF endorsement process but failed to gain endorsement, AQA adoption was rescinded. Although AQA focuses broadly on the three issues of performance measurement, data aggregation, and reporting, one of its key goals was to reach consensus on a set of physician-level quality measures that could be used by government purchasers or to guide private health insurance plan contracting decisions. This should help ultimately to standardize the performance measures used to assess and evaluate physician performance. AQA has now shifted its focus to identifying how quality measures are being used and implemented, as well as assessing where gaps exist in extant quality measures.

AQA-adopted measures may be used by CMS in its Physician Quality Reporting Initiative (PQRI), and many AQA-adopted measures were also used in PQRI's predecessor program, the Physician Voluntary Reporting Program (PVRP). For the 2009 PQRI, the measures meet one of the four following criteria:

- they are measures that were selected from the 2008 measure set,
- they are NQF-endorsed measures,
- they are AQA-adopted measures, or
- they were not NQF-endorsed or AQA-adopted at the time the proposed rule was published by CMS, but received endorsement or adoption by August 31, 2008.[32]

This allowed for a mechanism whereby measures were able to be implemented by CMS's PQRI without NQF endorsement, since AQA is recognized as a "consensus organization per section 1848(k)(2)(B) of the (Social Security) Act."[33] Given the lengthiness of NQF 's endorsement process, the large number of quality measures needing to go through the process, and AQA's recognized status as a consensus organization under law, AQA adoption allowed for expedited implementation of physician measures. As one commenter notes, this highlights a major challenge and tension inherent in the development and implementation of quality measures: "balancing the need for scientifically sound development processes against the need to have measures available for use."[34]

Selection and Implementation of Quality Measures

Once quality measures have been developed and ideally received endorsement, they will be considered for use in various quality activities. Since quality activities have varying goals (e.g., accountability, quality improvement) and are conducted in different settings for a variety of purposes, the selection stage is critical. This stage is especially consequential if the measures are being used for purposes of accountability, so the processes used by CMS to select measures for its pay-for-reporting programs (as part of its value-based purchasing initiative), and by CMS and other stakeholders for public reporting, are of particular import. The criteria used by CMS to select measures for its PQRI and RHQDAPU programs are discussed in more detail below.

AQA has also played a prominent role in the measure selection stage for physician measures. The AQA encourages and facilitates health plans and physicians to collaborate in determining which quality measures developed by the PCPI or the NCQA should be recommended for implementation. These recommendations are directed primarily to CMS for measure inclusion in its PQRI program, but also to smaller private payers for use in pay-for-performance programs. In this way, AQA contributes to prioritizing measures for implementation.

The following sections describe details of selected examples of implementation, specifically the Physician Quality Reporting Initiative (PQRI) and the Reporting Hospital Quality Data for Annual Payment Update (RHQDAPU) Program.

Physician Quality Reporting Initiative (PQRI)

The establishment of a quality reporting system for physicians was required by section 101(b) of the Tax Relief and Health Care Act of 2006 (TRHCA, P.L. 109-432), which also outlined a process for arriving at eligible quality measures. In response, CMS established the Physician Quality Reporting Initiative (PQRI) and began collecting physician-level quality data in July of 2007. PQRI was modeled on the Physician Voluntary Reporting Program (PVRP), which enabled physicians to voluntarily report quality data to CMS with no payment incentives, allowing the agency to establish a sound reporting infrastructure.

Unlike the PVRP, PQRI is a pay-for-reporting system and includes financial incentives for participation. Section 101(c) of TRHCA provided for financial incentives for the PQRI program and allowed for the awarding of an incentive payment to physicians based on the reporting of certain quality measures to begin in 2007. PQRI was extended for 2008 and 2009 by the Medicare, Medicaid, and SCHIP Extension Act of 2007 (MMSEA, P.L. 110-173) and was made permanent by the Medicare Improvements for Patients and Providers Act of 2008 (MIPPA, P.L. 110-275), which also allowed for incentive payments to continue through 2010.

The 2009 PQRI measure set contains more than 150 measures, and physicians are awarded a bonus payment of 2.0% of total allowed Physician Fee Schedule charges for covered professional services if they meet specified quality-reporting requirements. Measure reporting is either claims based or registry based,[35] and physicians may choose to report either on specific measures groups designated by CMS or on a series of unrelated measures, of the physician's choosing, that apply to their patient population.[36] The quality information collected through the PQRI program is not available to the public.

As noted previously, the quality measures included in the 2009 PQRI measure set were measures that either were included in the 2008 set, were NQF-endorsed, were AQA-adopted, or were undergoing consideration by either AQA or NQF for either adoption or endorsement. CMS identified six criteria that it employed when considering a measure for inclusion in its 2009 PQRI program. These include whether measures

- satisfy statutory requirements for selection (i.e., the measure was developed using a consensus-based process);
- are functional (i.e., useable);
- increase opportunities for eligible professionals to participate in the program or apply to an area without applicable measures;
- align with other CMS program health care goals;
- support CMS priorities (e.g., prevention, chronic conditions, high-cost and high-volume conditions, improved care coordination); and
- address various aspects of clinical care, including process, outcome, structure or patient experience.[37]

In addition, CMS takes the public comments received during the rulemaking process, and in response to other informal requests for input, into account when selecting measures for the PQRI program.

Reporting Hospital Quality Data for Annual Payment Update (RHQDAPU)

The development of the Reporting Hospital Quality Data for Annual Payment Update (RHQDAPU) program, as statutorily directed by Section 501(b) of the Medicare Prescription Drug, Improvement, and Modernization Act of 2003 (MMA, P.L. 108-173), represented one of CMS's early steps in the area of value-based purchasing. The RHQDAPU program requires participating hospitals to report specific quality data to CMS in order to receive a full annual payment update. Participation is voluntary, and hospitals may withdraw at any time.

The Deficit Reduction Act of 2005 (DRA, P.L. 109-171), Section 5001(a), provided for the continuation of this reporting requirement, and increased the at-risk percentage of the annual payment update from 0.4% to 2.0%. This section also required the Secretary to make the collected facility-specific quality data public.

The 2009 RHQDAPU measure set (for determining FY2010 payment) contains more than 40 measures and includes process measures; patient perspectives (through the HCAHPS, or Hospital Consumer Assessment of Healthcare Providers and Systems, survey); outcomes measures (30-day mortality rates); 30-day hospital readmission rates; selected AHRQ patient safety indicators (PSIs) and inpatient quality indicators (IQIs), three of which are composite measures; one measure assessing participation in a clinical registry; and one nursing-sensitive measure. The data reported and collected encompass several conditions identified as common in the Medicare population, including acute myocardial infarction, heart failure, and pneumonia, and also address surgical care improvement.

CMS has continually expanded the measure set used in its RHQDAPU program, building on the initial "starter set" of 10 measures, as directed by statute.[38] Initial expansion was guided by a baseline set of measures developed by the IOM and presented in its report "Performance Measurement: Accelerating Improvement." These measures included a number of Hospital Quality Alliance (HQA) measures, several structural measures, and the HCAHPS survey.[39] Established in 2002 by the Federation of American Hospitals (FAH), the American Association of Medical Colleges (AAMC), and the American Hospital Association (AHA), HQA has recommended hospital quality measures much as AQA adopted physician measures. HQA also collects and publishes quality information in partnership with CMS, although there is not perfect overlap between the HQA and RHQDAPU measure sets. The HQA has played an important role in adopting and implementing hospital quality measures, often adopting measures ahead of CMS and in this way allowing for informal user testing prior to adoption by CMS.

In addition to statutory requirements, the selection of measures for inclusion in the RHQDAPU program is guided by a series of six specific goals. These include

- expanding measures beyond process measures, to measures of outcome, patient perspectives, and efficiency;
- expanding the scope of hospital services to which the measures apply;
- considering the burden on hospitals;
- harmonizing the measures with other CMS quality programs;
- weighing the relevance and utility of the measures compared to the burden on hospitals; and
- using measures that are based on currently reported data (i.e., to clinical data registries or all-payer claims databases) or that do not require chart abstraction.[40]

CMS also prioritizes measures that evaluate high-burden, high-volume and high-cost conditions in the Medicare population and conditions (with established clinical guidelines) that persist in demonstrating wide variation in treatment and cost.[41] As it does when selecting measures for inclusion in PQRI, CMS also considers public comments it receives pursuant to the rulemaking process when selecting measures for the RHQDAPU program.

SELECTED ISSUES

The complexity of quality measurement, and the importance of its potential applications, has generated a number of policy and technical issues in terms of both measure development and implementation. Especially in the context of health care reform, these issues may be useful to consider as Congress develops policies aimed at improving health care quality. Some of these issues are discussed in more detail below.

Policy Issues

Perhaps the most commonly raised issue with respect to measuring, and therefore reporting, quality is the lack of harmonization of reporting requirements. Many reporting entities (physicians or hospitals, for example) report different quality measures to different entities for different purposes, and the burden and cost associated with this effort can be high. Efforts at streamlining requirements have been initiated, for example, by The Joint Commission and CMS; however, reporting requirements still tend to be complicated and laborious, as well as fairly costly. In addition, reporting entities may not always be provided with timely and useful feedback on their performance, decreasing the potential utility of the activity.

As noted previously in this chapter, a lack of standardized quality measures, and the lack of a uniform approach to generating these measures, have presented both challenges and opportunities. The diversity of stakeholders involved in the quality-measurement enterprise has resulted in a high degree of innovation in terms of measuring quality and related activities. It has also allowed practices to be developed that best suit a particular setting (e.g., hospitals) or purpose (e.g., accreditation). However, it has also created challenges with respect to the development of a set of measures that apply uniformly across all clinical areas and conditions, and this has resulted in a situation where measures may be unavailable to assess certain areas, or where only measures of questionable quality may be available. Measure gap areas include, for example, end-of-life care.

These measure gap areas may also result from a lack of evidence-based clinical guidelines in a particular clinical area or for a specific clinical condition. In these cases, in order to meet expedited policy goals, measures may be developed using consensus-based guidelines. While this has the benefit of facilitating measurement, it may also result in less robust quality measures in some cases.

Technical Issues

From a technical perspective, there are numerous issues that would ideally be addressed in order to achieve a robust quality measurement system. These issues may be divided into those that address validity and those that address reliability.

With respect to validity—that is, ensuring that quality measures are in fact measuring what they are intended to measure—a number of issues are critical. These include the proliferation of generally similar, yet slightly different, quality measures that could be used to measure the same process, structure, or outcome. For example, a search of AHRQ's National Quality Measures Clearinghouse (NQMC) identifies 10 quality measures related to receiving mammograms. This not only increases the burden of reporting on reporting entities, but also creates challenges with respect to drawing valid comparisons between measures. The problem of multiple similar measures is partially mitigated both by endorsement of measures and by the NQMC itself, which provides a uniform mechanism for comparing measures.

Issues with respect to accurate attribution—assigning the provision of a service to a specific physician or group practice—can make assessing quality of care challenging. Patients see multiple providers, which can complicate attributing processes to either a single encounter or provider. Issues of attribution may be alleviated, at least in part, by collecting patients' reports on the care they receive.

Finally, it can be difficult to link performance on outcome measures directly to the actions of providers. Health outcomes are influenced by a variety of variables that are not under the direct control of either the health care provider or the health care system, including environmental factors, access to health care services, and genetics. In addition, even though process and outcome are generally accepted to have a tighter linkage, issues have recently been raised regarding this relationship as well. In particular, it has been unclear whether strong performance on process of care measures is linked to decreased mortality rates. There is some evidence that in fact this relationship is not as tightly linked as it was believed to be.[42]

Ensuring reliability—that is, that measured results are consistent across repeated measurements— can also be technically challenging. Data sources must be appropriate and complete, as well as comparable across settings. Sample size (in this case, opportunities to provide "measured" care or to treat specified conditions for which outcomes are being measured) must be large enough to allow for drawing valid inferences about the performance of a single organization, a single provider within an organization, or a particular racial or ethnic group. Finally, standardization of quality measures is necessary in order to ensure that the same thing is being measured, according to the same specifications, across measurements.

CONCLUSION

The issue of improving the quality of health care is multifaceted, and policy makers have offered numerous approaches to addressing this policy problem. Measuring the quality of care delivered has served as the basis for a number of policy options being considered, but the effectiveness of these policy approaches depends on the quality of the data generated through measurement activities. The quality of this data in turn depends on the quality of the measure development process, as well as the way in which the measures are used and for what purpose. Congress may want to consider the issues outlined in this chapter when developing policy options that rely on quality measurement.

APPENDIX A. QUALITY MEASURE DEVELOPMENT PROCESSES (CMS, PCPI, AND NCQA)

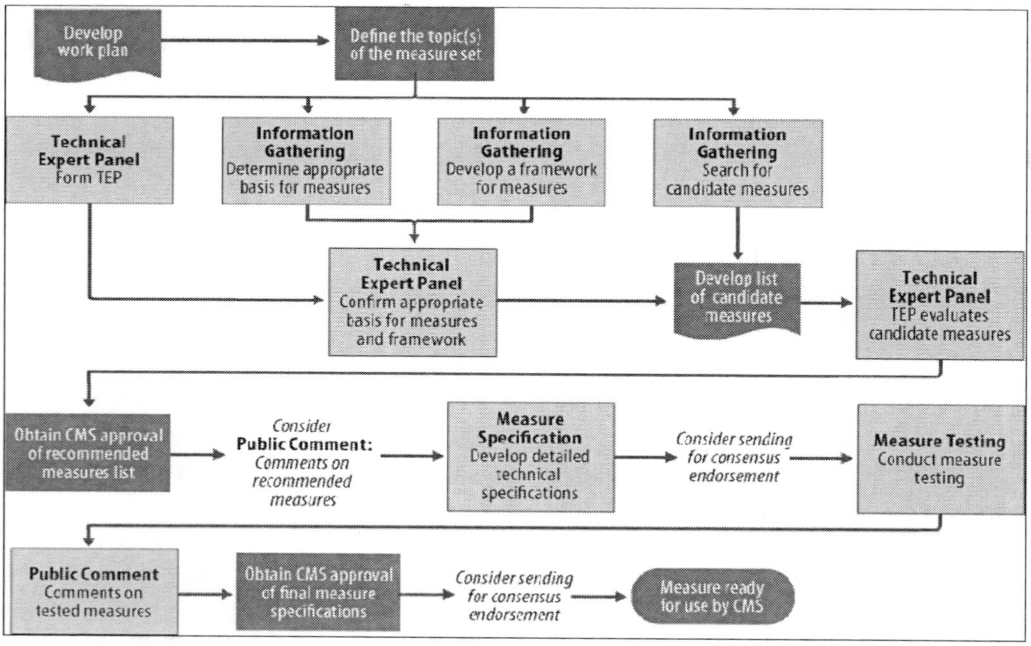

Source: CRS Adaptation from CMS's "Quality Measure Development Overview." Accessed at http://www.cms.hhs.gov/QualityInitiativesGenInfo/downloads/QualityMeasuresDevelopmentOverview.pdf.

Figure A- 1. CMS's Measure Development Process

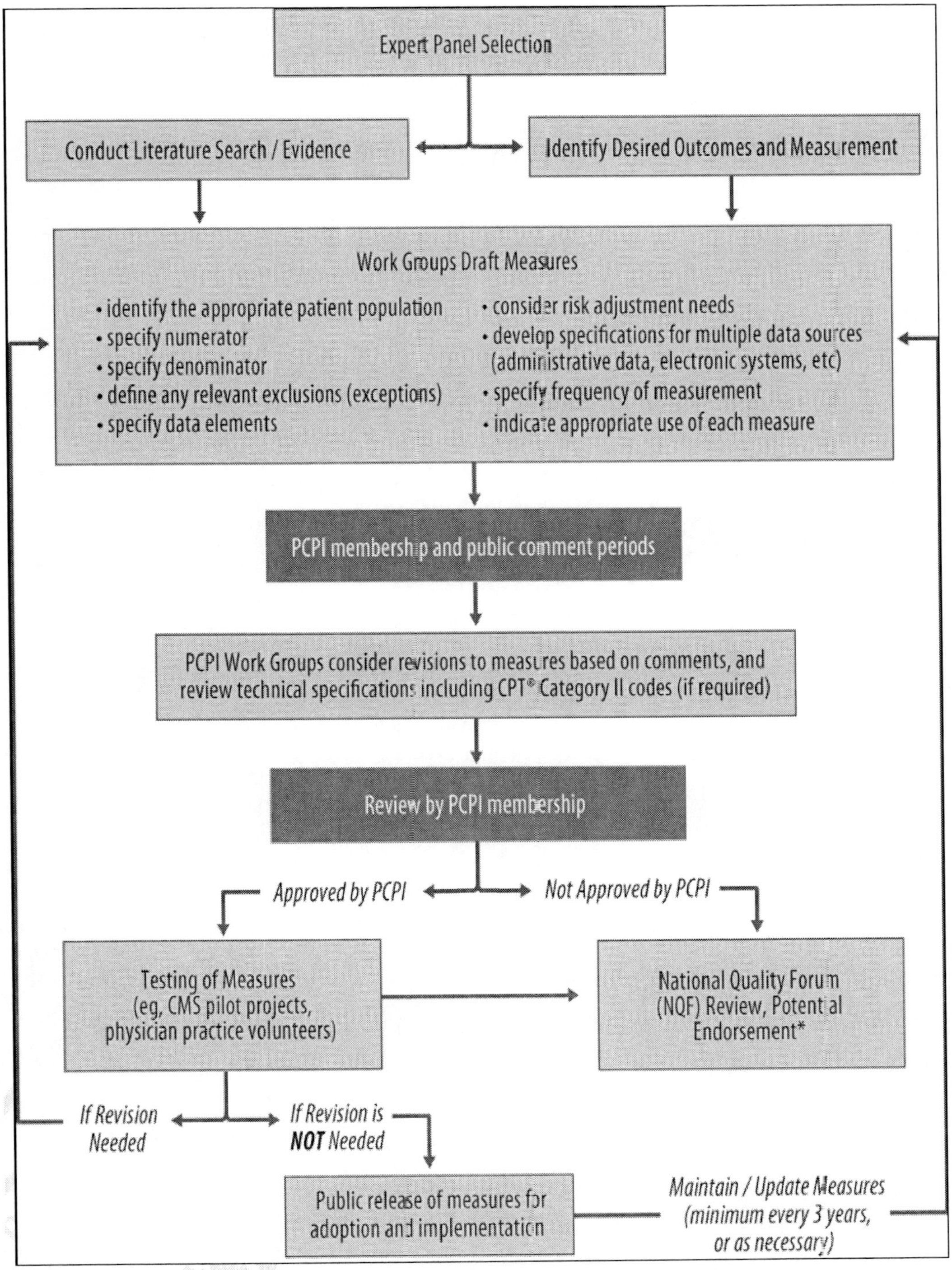

Source: CRS Adaptation from PCPI's "Measure Development Process."

Figure A-2. PCPI's Measure Development Process

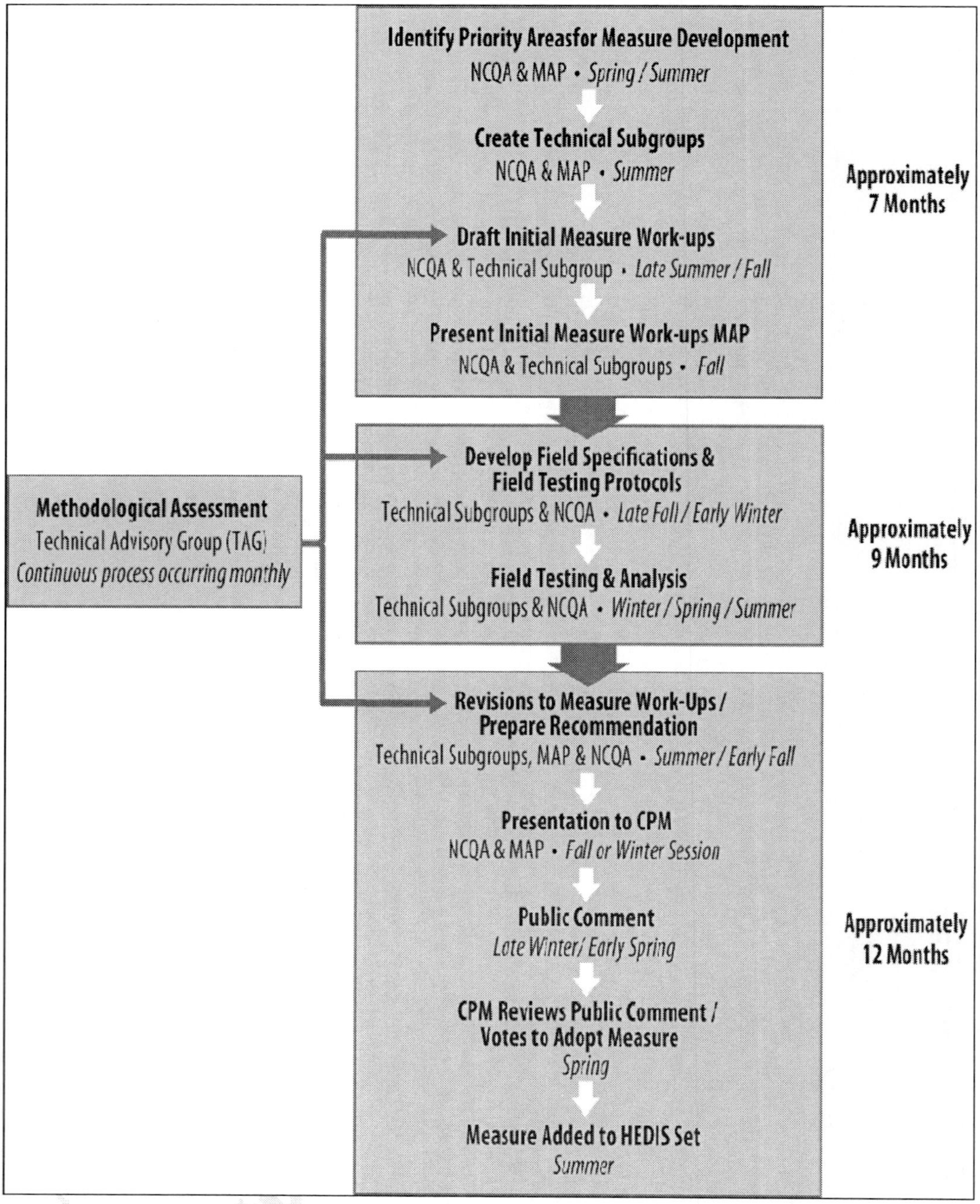

Source: CRS Adaptation from NCQA's "HEDIS Measure Development Process." Accessed at http://www.ncqa.org/Portals/0/HEDISQM/Measure_Development.pdf.

Figure A-3. NCQA's Measure Development Process

APPENDIX B. NQF'S MEASURE ENDORSEMENT PROCESS

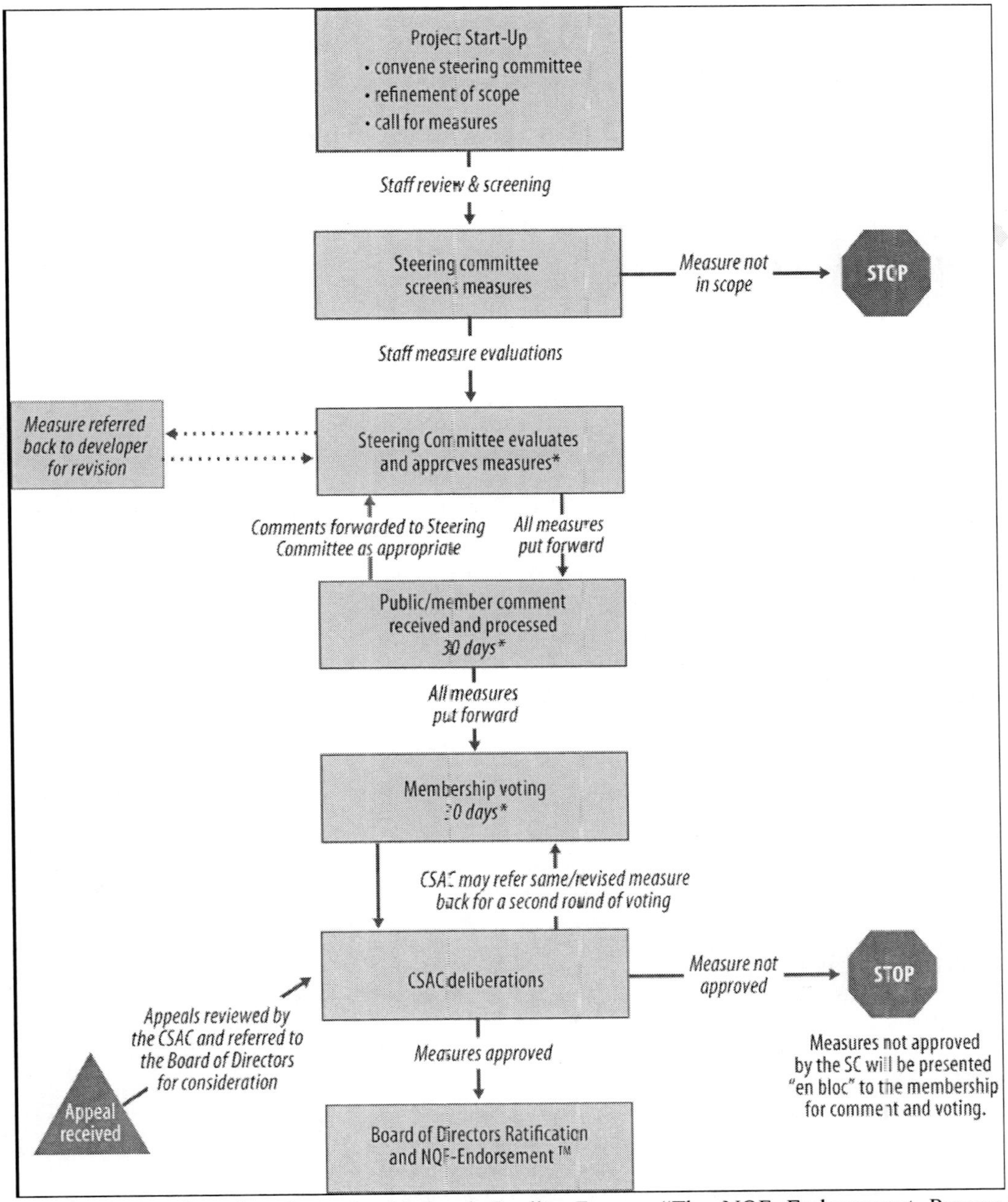

Source: CRS Adaptation from the National Quality Forum, "The NQF Endorsement Process." Accessed at http://www.qualityforum.org/ Publications/2008/10/The_NQF_Endorsement_Process.aspx.

Figure B-1. The Steps in the NQF Measure Endorsement Process

Appendix C. List of Acronyms

AAFP: American Academy of Family Physicians
ACP: American College of Physicians
AHIP: America's Health Insurance Plans
AHRQ: Agency for Healthcare Research and Quality
AMA: American Medical Association
AQA: The AQA Alliance
CMS: Centers for Medicare and Medicaid Services
HEDIS: Healthcare Effectiveness Data and Information Set
HQA: Hospital Quality Alliance
IOM: Institute of Medicine
OMB: Office of Management and Budget
NCQA: National Committee for Quality Assurance
NPP: National Priorities Partnership
NQF: National Quality Forum
PCPI: Physician Consortium for Performance Improvement
PQRI: Physician Quality Reporting Initiative
RHQDAPU: Reporting Hospital Quality Data for Annual Payment Update

End Notes

[1] Institute of Medicine (2001) "Crossing the Quality Chasm: A New Health System for the 21st Century," National Academy Press; Washington, DC; p. 1.

[2] Institute of Medicine (1999) "To Err is Human: Building a Better Health System." National Academy Press; Washington, D.C.

[3] Nolte, E., & McKee, C. M. (2008). "Measuring the health of nations: Updating an earlier analysis." Health Affairs, 27(1), 58-71. The conditions that are considered to be amenable to health care treatment include, but are not limited to, bacterial infections, treatable cancers, diabetes, cardiovascular and cerebrovascular disease, complications of common surgical procedures, and ischemic heart disease. The rate presented is an age-standardized death rate (SDR) per 100,000 population that is a simple average of the sex-specific SDRs, weighted for the distribution of males and females in the population.

[4] Midwest Business Group on Health. "Reducing the Costs of Poor-Quality Health Care Through Responsible Purchasing Leadership." April, 2003, pp. i-ii. http://www.mbgh.org/templates/UserFiles/Files/COPQ/copq%202nd%20printing.pdf.

[5] Schuster, M., McGlynn, E., & Brook, R. (1998). How good is the quality of health care in the United States? *Milbank Quarterly, 76,* 517-563.

[6] Mangione-Smith, R., Decristofaro, A. H., Setodji, C. M., Keesey, J., Klein, D. J., Adams, J. L., et al. (2007). The quality of ambulatory care delivered to children in the United States. *The New England Journal of Medicine, 26*(5), 644-649. E. A. McGlynn et al., "The Quality of Health Care Delivered to Adults in the United States", New England Journal of Medicine, 348(26), 2003

[7] Balas, E., Boren, A., Boren, S. (2000), "Managing clinical knowledge for health care improvement", Yearbook of Medical Informatics, pp. 65-70. National Library of Medicine, Bethesda, MD.

[8] Institute of Medicine. (2001) "Crossing the Quality Chasm: A New Health System for the 21st Century." National Academy Press; Washington D.C.; p. 232.

[9] A description of all of these activities is beyond the scope of this chapter. However, examples of quality research would include comparative effectiveness research, the development of clinical practice guidelines, or evidence syntheses. An example of quality measure development would include the development of the National Committee for Quality Assurance's Healthcare Effectiveness Data and Information Set (HEDIS) measures, and an example of quality reporting includes the Physician Quality Reporting Initiative (PQRI). Finally, examples of patient safety activity include the national level patient safety reporting system and nonpayment for "never events" policies.

[10] Donabedian, A. 1966. Evaluating the Quality of Medical Care. Milbank Memorial Fund Quarterly: Health and Society 44(3; pt. 2):166–203.

[11] The Agency for Healthcare Research and Quality (AHRQ). "Understanding Quality Measurement." Accessed at http://www.ahrq.gov/chtoolbx/understn.htm#domains.

[12] There are different types of composite measures, including appropriateness and opportunities measures. Appropriateness measures summarize performance across a group of measures related to a specific condition and require access to patient-level data. Opportunities measures are a basic summary across measures of opportunities for appropriate care, and are not reliant on patient-specific data, but rather may be calculated based on encounter data. AHRQ uses a number of composite measures in its National Healthcare Quality Report.

[13] Agency for Healthcare Research and Quality. "National Healthcare Quality Report 2008," at page 10. Accessed at http://www.ahrq.gov/qual/nhqr08/nhqr08.pdf on May 6, 2009.

[14] The National Quality Forum, a non-profit membership-based organization, aims to improve health care quality by setting national performance improvement priorities and endorsing quality measures.

[15] Section 1890(b)(1) of the Social Security Act.

[16] National Quality Forum. "Improving Healthcare Performance: Setting Priorities and Enhancing Measurement Capacity." Accessed at http://www.qualityforum.org/pdf/FINAL_2009NQFReporttoCongress.pdf on May 15, 2009.

[17] National Quality Forum. "NQF Time-Limited Endorsement." Accessed at http://www.qualityforum.org/pdf/txtime%20limited%20endorsement_csac_edits1 1-12-07.pdf on April 30, 2009.

[18] Accessed at http://www.jointcommission.org/NR/rdonlyres/D4B67088-980B-4642-A14F-ADB6805C1335/0/mktg_ahc.pdf on May 5, 2009.

[19] Riehle AI et al. (2007) "Specifying and Standardizing Performance Measures for Use at a National Level: Implications for Nursing-sensitive Care Performance Measures." *Medical Care Research and Review* 64(2):64S-8 1S at page 73S.

[20] NQF's measure evaluation criteria include whether a measure is linked to gains in quality and health outcomes; whether a measure is reliable and valid; whether a measure is usable (results are easy to understand and useful); and whether a measure is feasible (ease of access to required data). NCQA's desirable measure attributes include relevance; scientific soundness; and feasibility.

[21] Kmetik, K. (2007) "PCPI: What you should know about Consortium performance measures."*Current Clinical Practice* 1(1).

[22] CMS. "Quality Measures Development Overview." Accessed at http://www.cms.hhs.gov/ Quality Initiatives GenInfo/ downloads/QualityMeasuresDevelopmentOverview.pdf on May 14, 2009.

[23] CMS. "Roadmap for Quality Measurement in the Traditional Medicare Fee-for-Service Program." Accessed at http://www.cms.hhs.gov/QualityInitiativesGenInfo/downloads/QualityMeasuresDevelopmentOverview.pdf on May 14, 2009.

[24] PHS Act § 902(a); 42 U.S.C. § 299a.

[25] The Agency for Healthcare Research and Quality (AHRQ) maintains a public database of all health care quality measures, the National Quality Measures Clearinghouse (NQMC). Of the 1,762 measures currently in the database, 356 are NQF-endorsed. Accessed at http://www.qualitymeasures.ahrq.gov/ on April 28, 2009.

[26] Section 1 848(k)(2)(B)(i) of the Social Security Act.

[27] Section 1848(k)(2)(C)(i) of the Social Security Act. The contracting entity referred to here is the National Quality Forum. There is an exception provided in statute for cases where feasible and practical endorsed measures are not available in a specific clinical area. In these cases, the Secretary may specify a measure that is not endorsed. See section 1 848(k)(2)(C)(ii).

[28] Section 1886(b)(3)(B)(viii)(V) of the Social Security Act.

[29] Office of Management and Budget. Circular A-119. Accessed at http://www.whitehouse.gov/omb/circulars/a119/a1 19.html on April 30, 2009.

[30] 15 U.S.C. 272 note.

[31] National Quality Forum. "The NQF Endorsement Process." Accessed at http://www.qualityforum.org/pdf/factsheet_endorsement%20100908_FINAL.pdf on April 30, 2009.

[32] 73 *Federal Register* 69834 (November 19, 2008).

[33] 73 *Federal Register* 38566 (July 7, 2008).

[34] Riehle AI et al. (2007) "Specifying and Standardizing Performance Measures for Use at a National Level: Implications for Nursing-sensitive Care Performance Measures." *Medical Care Research and Review* 64(2):64S-8 1S at page 67S.

[35] Pilot testing of EHR-based reporting is currently underway for 10 of the 2009 measures, but incentive payments will not be based on measures submitted in this manner.

[36] CMS describes measure groups as being a group of at least four clinically-related measures that share a common denominator. The groups include diabetes mellitus, preventive care, chronic kidney disease, coronary artery bypass graft surgery, rheumatoid arthritis, back pain, and perioperative care. http://www.cms.hhs.gov/PQRI/15_MeasuresCodes.asp#TopOfPage, accessed May 20, 2009.

[37] 73 *Federal Register* 3 8566-7 (July 7, 2008).
[38] Section 1886(b)(3)(B)(viii)(IV) of the Social Security Act.
[39] This stage of expansion was statutorily mandated by Section 1886(b)(3)(B)(viii)(III) of the Social Security Act.
[40] CMS-1406-P, May 4, 2009, at page 335. Accessed at http://federalregister.gov/OFRUpload/OFRData/2009-10458_PI.pdf on May 20, 2009.
[41] Ibid.
[42] Werner RM and ET Bradlow. (2006) "Relationship Between Medicare's Hospital Compare Performance Measures and Mortality Rates." *JAMA* 296(22): 2694-2702.

Chapter 2

NATIONAL HEALTHCARE QUALITY REPORT-2009

Agency for Healthcare Research and Quality

ACKNOWLEDGMENTS

The NHQR is the product of collaboration among agencies across the Department of Health and Human Services (HHS). Many individuals guided and contributed to this chapter. Without their magnanimous support, this chapter would not have been possible.

Specifically, we thank:

Primary AHRQ Staff: Carolyn Clancy, William Munier, Katherine Crosson, Ernest Moy, and Karen Ho.

HHS Interagency Workgroup for the NHQR/NHDR: Girma Alemu (HRSA), Roxanne Andrews (AHRQ), Hakan Aykan (ASPE), Magda Barini-Garcia (HRSA), Douglas Boenning (HHS-ASPE), Miriam Campbell (CMS), Cecelia Casale (AHRQ-OEREP), Fran Chevarley (AHRQ-CFACT), Rachel Clement (HRSA), Agnes Davidson (OPHS), Denise Dougherty (AHRQ-OEREP), Erin Grace (AHRQ), Tanya Grandison (HRSA), Miryam Gerdine (OPHS-OMH), Darryl Gray (AHRQ-CQuIPS), Saadia Greenberg (AoA), Kirk Greenway (IHS), Karen Ho (AHRQ-CQuIPS), Edwin Huff (CMS), Kenneth Johnson (OCR), Jackie Shakeh Kaftarian (AHRQ-OEREP), Richard Klein (CDC-NCHS), Shari Ling (CMS), Leopold Luberecki (ASPE), Diane Makuc (CDC-NCHS), Ernest Moy (AHRQ-CQuIPS), Ryan Mutter (AHRQ), Karen Oliver (NIH-NIMH), Barry Portnoy (NIH/ODP), Georgetta Robinson (CMS), William Rodriguez (FDA), Rochelle Rollins (OMH), Asel Ryskulova (CDC-NCHS), Judy Sangl (AHRQ-CQuIPS), Adelle Simmons (HHS-ASPE), Alan E. Simon (CDC-NCHS), Sunil Sinha (CMS), Jane Sisk (CDC-NCHS), Nancy Sonnenfeld (CDC-NCHS), Caroline Taplin (HHS-ASPE), Karmen Todd (OCR), Benedict Truman (CDC), Joan Van Nostrand (HRSA), Valerie Welsh (OPHS-OMH), Odies Williams (OCR), and Deborah Willis-Fillinger (HRSA).

AHRQ NHQR/NHDR Team: Roxanne Andrews, Denise Burgess, Fran Chevarley, Cecilia Casale, Rita Coleman, Daniel Crespin, Katherine Crosson, Denise Dougherty, Darryl Gray, Karen Ho, Jackie Shakeh Kaftarian, Ernest Moy, William Munier, Ryan Mutter, Judy Sangl, and Marc Zodet.

HHS Data Experts: Umed Ajani (CDC), Roxanne Andrews (AHRQ), Frances Chevarley (AHRQ), Steven Cohen (AHRQ), James Colliver (SAMHSA), Paul Eggers (NIH-NIDDK), John Fleishman (AHRQ), Anita Gadzuk (SAMHSA), Joe Gfroerer (SAMHSA), Kirk Greenway (IHS), Stan Lehman (CDC), Robert Pratt (CDC), Valerie Robison (CDC), Beatrice Rouse (SAMHSA), Asel Ryskulova (CDC-NCHS), Alan E. Simon (CDC-NCHS), Jane Sisk (CDC-NCHS), Cheryll Thomas (CDC), Debra Trunzo (SAMHSA), and Marc Zodet (AHRQ).

Other Data Experts: Valarie Ashby (U-Michigan), Marguerite Barrett (Thomson Reuters), Dale Bratzler (Oklahoma QIO), Joachim Bruess (NCQA), Xiuhua Chen (SSS), Rosanna Coffey (Thomson Reuters), Stephen Connor (NHPCO), Maureen Curry (Qualidigm), Claudia Dahlerus (Qualidigm), Celia Dahlman (Fu Associates), Thomas Dudley (Qualidigm), Stephen Edge (Rosewell Park Cancer Institute), David Grant (UCLA), Michael Halpern (American Cancer Society), Matthew Haskins (NHPCO), Allen Ma (Oklahoma QIO), Lauren Miller (Oklahoma QIO), Wato Nsa (Oklahoma QIO), Bryan Palis (NCBD, American College of Surgeons), Royce Park (UCLA), Allison Petrilla (NHPCO), Mary Pratt (Qualidigm), John Rauch (Westat), Susan Reimann (U-Michigan), William Ross (Fu Associates), Robin Sands (U-Michigan), Carol Spence (NHPCO), Andrew Stewart (NCBD, American College of Surgeons), Elizabeth Ward (American Cancer Society), Mike Wilson (Westat), and Claudia Wright (Oklahoma QIO).

Other AHRQ Contributors: Barbara Barton, Doreen Bonnett, Cindy Brach, Celia Dahlman, Karen Fleming-Michael, William Freeman, Paul Gorrell, Biff LeVee, Morgan Liscinski, Corey Mackison, Kathy McKay, Gerri Michael-Dyer, Karen Migdail, Pamela Owens, Mamatha Pancholi, Larry Patton, Wendy Perry, Deborah Queenan, John Rauch, Mary Rolston, Scott Rowe, Randie Siegel, Christine Williams, Mike Wilson, and Phyllis Zucker.

Data Support Contractors: CHD-Fu, Social and Scientific Systems, Thomson Reuters Healthcare, and Westat.

HIGHLIGHTS

Key Themes and Highlights from the National Healthcare Quality Report

Health care seeks to diagnose, treat, and improve the physical and mental well-being of all Americans. Across the lifespan, health care helps people stay healthy, recover from illness, live with chronic disease or disability, and cope with death and dying. Quality health care delivers these services in a way that is safe, timely, patient centered, efficient, and equitable.[1] Unfortunately, Americans too often do not receive care that they need, or they receive care that causes harm. Care can also be delivered too late or without full consideration of a patient's preferences and values. Many times, our system of health care distributes services inefficiently and unevenly across populations.

Each year since 2003, the Agency for Healthcare Research and Quality (AHRQ), together with its partners in the Department of Health and Human Services (HHS), has reported on progress and opportunities for improving health care quality, as mandated by the U.S. Congress. The information amassed for the National Healthcare Quality Report (NHQR) since its inception is a growing knowledge base that can be used to address three critically important questions:

- What is the status of health care quality in the United States?
- Where is health care quality improvement most needed?
- How is the quality of the health care delivered to Americans changing over time?

The significance of tracking this sector's performance is evident from many vantage points. More than $2 trillion is spent each year on health care in the United States.[2] Spending on health care is escalating relentlessly, threatening the financial security of families and businesses. Quality and value are increasingly considered in the decisions patients and payers make. To help patients choose doctors and hospitals prudently, tools have been produced that gather information about hospitals and rate health care providers. To motivate providers to deliver high-quality care, some purchasers reward superior performance. In addition, some refuse to pay for additional care needed to correct hospital-acquired conditions that could reasonably have been prevented through the application of evidence-based medicine. Monitoring the success of these efforts is crucial to help stakeholders refine quality improvement activities and to lead Americans toward the optimal health care they need and deserve.

The NHQR is built on more than 200 measures categorized across four dimensions of quality: effectiveness, patient safety, timeliness, and patient centeredness. Guided by a subcommittee of AHRQ's National Advisory Council and an HHS Interagency Work Group,[I] the NHQR focuses on a group of core report measures that represent the most important and scientifically credible measures of quality for the Nation. By focusing on core measures, the NHQR provides a readily understandable summary and explanation of the key results derived from available data.

Three themes from the 2009 NHQR emphasize the need to accelerate progress if the Nation is to achieve higher quality health care in the near future:

- Health care quality needs to be improved, particularly for uninsured individuals, who are less likely to get recommended care.
- Some areas merit urgent attention, including patient safety and health care-associated infections (HAIs).
- Quality is improving, but the pace is slow, especially for preventive care and chronic disease management.

We also summarize AHRQ and HHS efforts to accelerate the pace of improvement by:

- Improving measurement.
- Removing barriers to quality care.
- Empowering providers with health information technology (HIT) and training.
- Establishing and sustaining partnerships to lead change.

Health Care Quality Needs to be Improved, Particularly for Uninsured Individuals, Who Are Less Likely to Get Recommended Care

The key function of the NHQR is to summarize the state of health care quality for the Nation. This undertaking is difficult, as no single national health care quality survey collects a standard set of data elements from the same defined population for the same period each year. Rather, data come from a wide range of sources that focus on different populations and data years.

Despite the data limitations, we find that health care quality in America is suboptimal. The gap between best possible care and that which is routinely delivered remains substantial across the Nation. Receipt of quality health care also varies widely. For example, caregivers reported that 95% of hospice patients received the right amount of pain medication, but only 8% of patients needing care for alcohol problems received such treatment at a specialty facility. Across the core report measures tracked in the NHQR, the median level of receipt of needed services was 58%. We can and should do better.

Moreover, despite efforts to transform the U.S. health care system to focus on effective preventive and chronic illness care, it continues to perform better when delivering diagnostic and therapeutic care in response to acute medical problems. Our system achieves higher performance on hospital measures, such as acute treatment for heart attacks, than on outpatient measures, such as cancer screening and diabetes management. For example, between the 2008 and 2009 reports, five measures attained overall performance levels exceeding 95%.[II] Four of these five measures relate to hospital care for heart attack. In addition, all 10 of the worst performing process measures tracked in this NHQR are measures of outpatient care, and 6 of these relate to preventive services.

For individuals without health insurance, quality of care is even worse. For many years, the National Healthcare Disparities Report (NHDR) has examined disparities in care related to insurance. In this NHQR, we report on the relationship between uninsurance and quality of care. Insurance status of individuals could be identified for 35 process measures the NHQR tracks.[III] Across these measures, the median level of receipt of services was 50% among uninsured individuals compared with 65% among privately insured individuals.

Table 1 shows the 10 measures with the largest difference between individuals with private insurance and those with no insurance. Individuals age 65 and over are excluded because almost all have Medicare. Also, these data do not reflect the current economic recession, which may exacerbate insurance-related differences in care.

Uninsured people are less likely to get recommended care for disease prevention and management (Table H.1). Large differences were observed between individuals with private insurance and no insurance for measures related to:

- Preventive services, including cancer screening, dental care, counseling about diet and exercise, and flu vaccination.
- Diabetes management.

Table H.2 shows the 10 measures with the smallest differences between individuals with private insurance and no insurance. Uninsured individuals are only slightly less likely to receive counseling about booster seats and passive smoking; adequate time with health providers; pneumococcal vaccination; and appropriate breast cancer treatment. Uninsured and privately insured individuals are about equally likely to have discussions with their regular doctors about medications and treatments from other doctors and to receive care related to HIV disease.

Table H.1. Measures with Largest Differences between Individuals with Private Insurance and no Insurance

Measure	Private insurance (%)	No insurance (%)	Difference (Private - No insurance)
Women ages 40-64 who had a mammogram in the last 2 years	74.2	38.3	35.9
Children ages 2-17 who had a dental visit in the calendar year	59.6	27.9	31.7
Adults ages 40-64 with diagnosed diabetes who received a dilated eye examination in the calendar year	64.1	35.4	28.7
Adults ages 50-64 who ever received a colonoscopy, sigmoidoscopy, or proctoscopy	47.5	20.7	26.8
Adults ages 18-64 with obesity who received advice from a provider to exercise	61.0	41.2	19.8
Women ages 18-64 who received a Pap smear in the last 3 years	86.3	66.9	19.4
Adults ages 40-64 with diagnosed diabetes who received a hemoglobin A1c measurement in the calendar year	94.2	75.7	18.5
Adults ages 18-64 with obesity who received advice about healthy eating	50.3	32.0	18.3
Children ages 2-17 who received advice about healthy eating	59.1	41.4	17.7
Adults ages 18-64 at high risk (e.g., diabetes) who received an influenza vaccination in the last 12 months	32.5	16.8	15.7

Note: All differences in this table are statistically significant.

Table H.2. Measures with Smallest Differences between Individuals with Private Insurance and no Insurance

Measure	Private insurance (%)	No insurance (%)	Difference (Private - No insurance)
Children who weigh 41-80 pounds for whom a health provider ever gave advice about using booster seats when riding in a car	46.4	41.7	4.7
Children who had a doctor's office or clinic visit in the last 12 months whose health providers spent enough time with them	94.5	91.5	3.0
Adults ages 18-64 at high risk (e.g., COPD*) who ever received pneumococcal vaccination	16.8	14.2	2.6
Women under age 65 treated for breast cancer with breast-conserving surgery who received radiation therapy within 1 year of diagnosis	76.0	73.6	2.4
Patients under age 65 with colon cancer who received surgical resection of colon cancer that included at least 12 lymph nodes pathologically examined	69.8	68.2	1.6
Women under age 65 with Stage I-IIb breast cancer who received axillary node dissection or sentinel lymph node biopsy at the time of surgery (lumpectomy or mastectomy)	91.2	90.0	1.2
Children for whom a health provider ever gave advice about how smoking in the house can be bad for a child	43.1	42.7	0.4
People under age 65 with a usual source of care who usually asks about prescription medications and treatments from other doctors	79.4	79.5	-0.1
Adult patients with HIV and CD4 count <50 who received *Mycobacterium avium* complex prophylaxis	91.3	91.8	-0.5
Adult patients with HIV and CD4 count <200 who received *Pneumocystis* pneumonia prophylaxis	93.9	94.8	-0.9

Note: None of the differences in this table are statistically significant.
*COPD=chronic obstructive pulmonary disease

For almost all measures, uninsured people were less likely to receive recommended care compared with privately insured people. As shown in the tables, gaps were particularly large for preventive care and diabetes management and smaller gaps were observed for cancer treatment. Cancer is typically treated in hospitals and associated outpatient facilities that may be more able and committed to providing charity care. The Ryan White HIV/AIDS Program, which provides HIV-related services to individuals who are uninsured or unable to afford these services, may help explain why uninsured patients receive HIV care similar in quality to privately insured patients. In addition, uninsured patients may be more willing to pay out of pocket for treatment of cancer or HIV disease than for preventive services.

Some Areas Merit Urgent Attention, Including Patient Safety and Health Care-Associated Infections

After determining that quality is suboptimal, the next step toward improvement, and the second key function of the NHQR, is to identify which areas are in greatest need of intervention. Potential problem areas can be defined in terms of types of services and geography. In this section, we focus on one aspect of care that is performing particularly poorly: patient safety. Then, we examine some areas of the country where performance is lagging.

Patient Safety

Improvement is important across all dimensions of health care quality. It is critically important in the area of patient safety. Patients have a reasonable expectation that they will not be harmed by the health care they receive. For more than 6 years, the NHQR has presented a summary of the safety of health care provided to the American people.

Tracking trends in patient safety is complicated by difficulties assessing and ensuring the systematic reporting of medical errors and patient safety events. However, with improvements in data quality and methods, a clearer picture of trends in health care safety is emerging. In previous reports, we used the most recent data year compared with a baseline data year to calculate rate of change. This year, we introduced a new methodology for quantifying change by entering estimates for all available data years into a regression model to calculate rate of change. In addition, we retired measures that have achieved a rate of 95% or higher. We believe these changes yield more stable and robust estimates of rate of change.

Analysis of patient safety has been based on a set of databases that were created in response to the need for information documented in such publications as the Institute of Medicine's landmark 2000 report *To Err Is Human: Building a Safer Health System*.[3] Some of our findings are disturbing. For example, last year we reported that approximately one out of seven adult hospitalized Medicare patients experienced one or more adverse events. This year, we see problems specifically in the area of HAIs.

- **In hospitals, safety remains a significant problem.** Of the 33 hospital measures related to safety, 12 (36%) improved at a rate greater than 5% per year (Figure H.1). In contrast, of the 19 hospital measures not related to safety, 16 (84%) improved at a rate greater than 5% per year. Still, more than half of safety measures showed some improvement.

Health Care-Associated Infections

Infections acquired during hospital care, also known as nosocomial infections, are one of the most serious patient safety concerns. It is unfortunate that HAI rates are not declining. Of all the measures in the NHQR measure set, the one worsening at the fastest rate is postoperative sepsis (Table H.3). The two process measures related to HAIs tracked in the NHQR, both covering timely receipt of prophylactic antibiotics for surgery, are improving steadily. However, HAI outcome measures are lagging; only one shows improvement over time while three are worsening and one shows no change. This may, in part, reflect improving detection of HAIs.

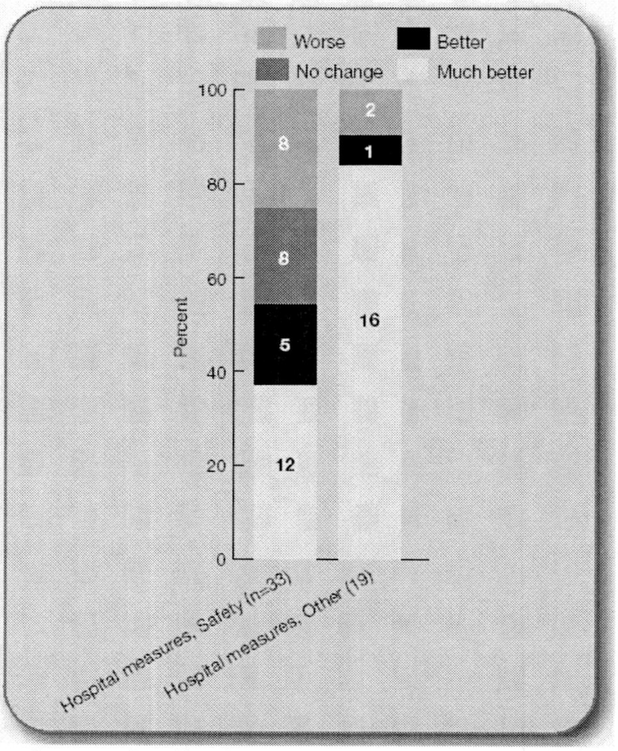

Worse = Quality is going in a negative direction at an average annual rate greater than 1% per year.
No Change = Quality is not changing or is changing at an average annual rate less than 1% per year.
Better = Quality is going in a positive direction at an average annual rate between 1% and 5% per year.
Much Better = Quality is going in a positive direction at an average annual rate greater than 5% per year.
Note: Go to Chapter 1, Introduction and Methods, for discussion of year intervals used for analysis. N indicates number of measures included in each group

Figure H.1. Change in hospital quality over time, safety measures versus other hospital measures

It is evident that more attention devoted to patient safety is needed to ensure that health care does not result in avoidable patient harm. Systems for identifying and learning from patient safety events need to be improved. Patient safety reporting systems are often laborious and cumbersome, and health care providers express fear that findings may be used against them in court or harm their professional reputations. Many factors, such as concerns about sharing confidential data across facilities or State lines, limit the ability to aggregate data in sufficient numbers to rapidly identify important risks and hazards in the delivery of patient care. More work is also needed to develop measures that capture the underlying processes and conditions that lead to adverse events and the practices that are most effective in mitigating them.

Fortunately, recent progress has been made in raising awareness, improving event reporting systems, and establishing national standards for data collection. The Patient Safety and Quality Improvement Act of 2005 provides for the voluntary formation of Patient Safety Organizations (PSOs). Under this legislation, these entities can receive and analyze patient safety data and work with providers to improve care without fear of legal discovery. PSOs also can report deidentified data to a Network of Patient Safety Databases, and findings from this resource will be published in future NHQRs and NHDRs. Currently, 69 organizations have been listed by HHS as PSOs.

Table H.3. Measures of Health Care-Associated Infections, Annual Rates of Improvement

	Annual rate of improvement (%)	Data source
Process Measures		
Adult surgery patients who received prophylactic antibiotics within 1 hour prior to surgical incision	26.4	QIO
Adult surgery patients who had prophylactic antibiotics discontinued within 24 hours after surgery end time	32.9	QIO
Outcome Measures		
Adult surgery patients with postoperative pneumonia	11.6	MPSMS
Bloodstream infections associated with central venous catheter placements	No change	MPSMS
Selected infections due to medical care	-1.6	HCUP
Adult surgery patients with postoperative catheter-associated urinary tract infection	-3.6	MPSMS
Postoperative sepsis	-8.0	HCUP

Key: QIO = Centers for Medicare & Medicaid Services (CMS) Quality Improvement Organization Program; MPSMS = CMS Medicare Patient Safety Monitoring System; HCUP = AHRQ Healthcare Cost and Utilization Project Nationwide Inpatient Sample.

Note: Annual rate of improvement is calculated from regression models using all available data years. Positive values indicate increased rates of recommended processes of care or decreased rates of adverse events. Negative values indicate increased rates of adverse events. No change indicates rate changed by less than 1% per year. MPSMS includes adult Medicare beneficiaries only; QIO and HCUP include all payers.

The Patient Safety and Quality Improvement Act also addresses an issue that has plagued data collection related to patient safety: the lack of standardized vocabularies that ensure a common definition of specific terms.[4] AHRQ coordinated the development of common definitions and reporting formats for patient safety events. The beta version of the Common Formats was released in 2008 and supports data aggregation, analysis, and learning throughout the quality improvement cycle. The National Quality Forum (NQF) then solicited feedback from private-sector organizations and convened an expert panel to provide recommendations to AHRQ. The revised Common Formats Version 1.0 was subsequently released in September 2009.

Geographic Variation

Quality of care varies not only across types of care but also across geographic areas. Knowing where to focus efforts improves the efficiency of interventions. Delivering data that can be used for local benchmarking and improvement is a key step in raising awareness and driving quality improvement. AHRQ's State Snapshots tool (http://statesnapshots.ahrq.gov) was launched in 2005. This Web site helps State health leaders, researchers, consumers, and others understand the status of health care quality in individual States and the District of

Columbia. The State Snapshots are based on more than 100 NHQR measures, each of which evaluates a different aspect of health care performance and shows each State's strengths and weaknesses.

Although we observe wide variation across States, those in the upper Midwest and New England tend to achieve the highest overall quality of care while States in the Southwest and South Central parts of the country tend to have the lowest quality and may benefit from more urgent attention. Although the measures are often the products of complex statistical formulas, results are expressed on the Web site as simple, five-color graphic "performance meters." The State Snapshots also allow users to compare a State's performance with that of other States in the same region and to see how a State compares with best performing States.

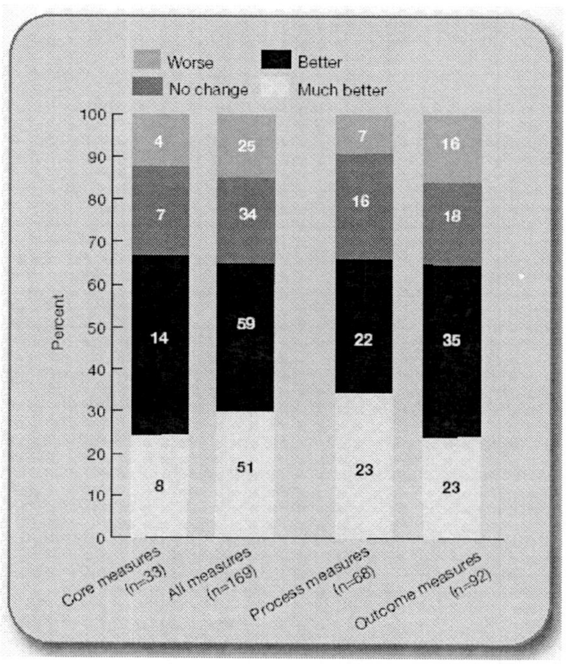

Worse = Quality is going in a negative direction at an average annual rate greater than 1% per year.
No Change = Quality is not changing or is changing at an average annual rate less than 1% per year.
Better = Quality is going in a positive direction at an average annual rate between 1% and 5% per year.
Much Better = Quality is going in a positive direction at an average annual rate greater than 5% per year.
Note: Go to Chapter 1, Introduction and Methods, for discussion of year intervals used for analysis. N indicates number of measures included in each group for which change could be measured over time.

Figure H.2. Change in quality over time

In addition to maps showing variation in quality of care, this NHQR introduces a new type of State map to help target interventions. These maps combine information about processes of care and associated outcomes. For example, we include a map that shows information about a process typically needed to keep the glucose level of patients with diabetes under control, receipt of hemoglobin A1c testing, and an outcome of poor control of glucose, hospitalizations for short-term complications, such as diabetic ketoacidosis. These maps do not imply causality because processes of care may not affect outcomes for many years. However, by linking related measures, we hope information in these maps will help motivate specific States to act. States with poor outcomes for which a specific performance issue has been identified may be well positioned to improve quality of care.

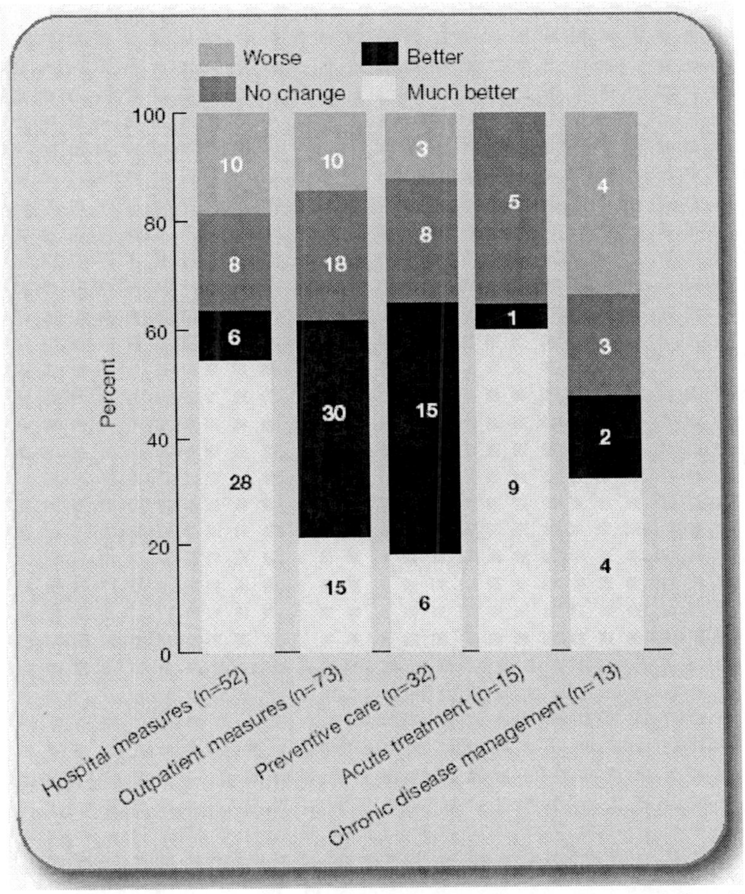

Worse = Quality is going in a negative direction at an average annual rate greater than 1% per year.

No Change = Quality is not changing or is changing at an average annual rate less than 1% per year.

Better = Quality is going in a positive direction at an average annual rate between 1% and 5% per year.

Much Better = Quality is going in a positive direction at an average annual rate greater than 5% per year.

Note: Go to Chapter 1, Introduction and Methods, for discussion of year intervals used for analysis. N indicates number of measures included in each group for which change could be measured over time.

Figure H.3. Change in quality over time by setting and type of measure

Quality is Improving, But the Pace is Slow, Especially in Preventive Care and Chronic Disease Management

Suboptimal quality of care is undesirable, but we may be less concerned if we observe evidence of vigorous improvement. Hence, the third key function of the NHQR is to examine change over time. To track the progress of health care quality in this country, the NHQR presents an annual rate of change in quality, which represents how quickly quality of services delivered by the health care system is improving or declining based on the report's measures. Another way to describe this is the speed of improvement or decline in the quality of the U.S. health care system.

- **Quality is improving at a slow pace.** Of the 33 core measures, two-thirds improved, 14 (42%) with a rate between 1% and 5% per year and 8 (24%) with a rate greater than 5% per year (Figure H.2). The median rate of change was 2% per year. Across all 169 measures, results were similar, although the median rate of change was slightly higher at 2.3% per year.
- **Process and outcome measures are improving.** Of the 68 process measures, 23 (34%) improved at a rate greater than 5% per year. Overall, the median rate of change was 2.2% per year. Improvement is somewhat slower for outcomes. Of the 92 outcome measures, 23 (25%) improved at a rate greater than 5% per year. Overall, the median rate of change was 2.3% per year.
- **Measures of hospital care improve more quickly than measures of outpatient care.** Of the 52 hospital measures, 28 (54%) improved at a rate greater than 5% per year (Figure H.3). The median rate of change was 5.8% per year. In contrast, of the 73 outpatient measures, only 15 (21%) improved at a rate greater than 5% per year. The median rate of change was 1.4% per year. Still, almost two-thirds of outpatient measures showed some improvement.
- **Measures of acute treatment improve more quickly than measures of preventive care and chronic disease management.** The three measure categories, preventive care, acute treatment, and chronic disease management, reflect different types of care that patients often need. The highest rate of improvement was in measures related to treatment. Of the 15 process of care measures related to treatment of acute illnesses or injuries, 9 (60%) improved at a rate greater than 5% per year. In contrast, of the 32 process measures related to preventive services, only 6 (19%) improved at a rate greater than 5% per year. Of the 13 process measures related to chronic disease management, only 4 (31%) improved at this higher rate. Still, two-thirds of preventive care measures and almost half of chronic disease management measures showed some improvement.

In the analysis of trends for this year's NHQR, it is clear that quality improvements continue to be unevenly spread across the settings of care. Some areas have shown increasing rates of improvement while improvements in other areas have slowed. For example, care delivered in hospitals improved at an annual rate of change of almost 6%, which continues to be the highest rate of quality improvement among the major health care delivery settings. In contrast, care in outpatient settings improved at a rate that only slightly exceeded 1%.

Significant improvement in hospital care has occurred since the Centers for Medicare & Medicaid Services (CMS) began reporting consensus-based quality measures on the Hospital Quality Compare Web site (http://www.hospitalcompare.hhs.gov). Of the 10 fastest improving measures tracked in the NHQR, 8 were measures published on the CMS Web site.

Similarly, improvement in preventive services and chronic disease management lagged behind improvement in acute disease treatment. Of the nine process measures tracked in the NHQR that got worse instead of better, four were preventive services, including mammography, Pap testing, and fecal occult blood testing. Four services were related to chronic disease management, including three services for patients with diabetes.

When examining change across types of care and care settings, it is often difficult to determine from the available data why changes in performance occur. Public reporting and strong advocacy from multiple stakeholders in support of quality, as in the case of CMS measures, may influence broad system change and subsequent quality improvements. Institutional health care settings, such as hospitals and nursing homes, are more likely to have structured quality improvement programs and staff that help raise performance in these organizations. Staff exert a high degree of influence over patient behaviors and the therapeutic milieu during a patient stay. The greater availability of HIT as part of institutional infrastructure may also contribute to improvements in quality in these settings. In contrast, doctors' offices often do not have sufficient resources, staff, and training to apply quality improvement techniques efficiently and rely upon patients to implement care recommendations.

Efforts Are Needed to Accelerate Improvement

This 2009 report summarizes areas where progress in health care quality has excelled and where it has lagged. But national reports do not improve quality by themselves. Measures need to be adapted to guide local interventions. Barriers to quality care, such as uninsurance, need to be overcome. Providers need to be empowered with HIT and training. Community partnerships that bring together all the stakeholders who can make or break a quality improvement initiative need to be created and maintained. Building on information contained in the NHQR and NHDR, HHS organizations are working on an exciting range of programs that seek to accelerate the pace of health care quality improvement nationwide.

Improve Measurement

New quality measures are needed. The complex nature of health care makes measuring the quality of health care services particularly difficult. As scientific evidence evolves, we must not only ensure revision and coordination of existing quality measures but also develop new quality measures to address emerging issues. For example, it is increasingly recognized that some aspects of quality can best be assessed when viewed through a patient's eyes. Patients see problems from a personal perspective and may observe deficiencies that busy providers do not notice. For example, they may be uniquely situated to detect flaws during transitions of care and experience the effects of inadequate care coordination. Patient centeredness, the aspect of quality related to patient self-management and engagement in medical decisionmaking, can only be defined from a patient's perspective. Measures from AHRQ's Consumer Assessment of Healthcare Providers and Systems (CAHPS®) surveys capture some aspects of patients' experiences with care, but more work is urgently needed to expand patient-focused measures of health care quality.

Healthy People (http://www.healthypeople.gov) provides science-based, 10-year national objectives for promoting health and preventing disease. Since 1979, Healthy People has measured and tracked national health objectives to encourage collaborations, guide individuals toward making informed health decisions, and assess the impact of prevention activity. Healthy People 2020 is currently under development. Through a national consensus process, it is identifying specific objectives for improving the health of the Nation, establishing baseline values for the objectives, and setting specific targets to be achieved by 2020. Overaching goals for Healthy People 2020 are: (1) Eliminate preventable disease, disability, injury, and premature death; (2) Achieve health equity, eliminate disparities, and improve the health of all groups; (3) Create social and physical environments that promote good health for all; and (4) Promote healthy development and healthy behaviors across every stage of life.

Measure sets need to be coordinated. Another challenge is the often opportunistic, incremental, and fragmented development of quality measures without detailed consideration of data sources, analysis and maintenance requirements, and user needs. Uncoordinated and isolated measure development can lead different groups to create and advocate competing and sometimes conflicting measures of the same process or outcome. At best, this is duplicative; at worst, it can create confusion, irritation, and unnecessary labor for providers trying to supply quality information to multiple stakeholders. Calls for new measures may also be hampered by resource constraints.[5, 6]

The work of the NQF helps to enhance measure harmonization and reduce measure clutter. Its mission is to coordinate and promote the consensus development process for health care quality measurement among its organizational members. NQF has endorsed more than 500 measures, and this library represents the best means currently available to track quality of care. What is needed now is consensus on a single set of core measures that all payers and stakeholders will use to monitor quality improvement. Such a set would facilitate benchmarking and reduce the measurement burden on providers.

Along with achieving consensus on a core measure set, systems for maintaining and revising this set are needed. The HHS Measure Inventory (available through the National Quality Measures Clearinghouse at http://www.qualitymeasures.ahrq.gov/hhs/hhs.index.aspx) is a step in this direction. Released in 2008, this tool provides specifications of measures that HHS uses for quality measurement, reporting, and improvement. It is designed to help synchronize measurement and advance collaboration within the quality improvement community toward a uniform set of performance measures.

Remove Barriers to Quality Care

Lack of health insurance is a major hindrance to quality care and should be reduced. As demonstrated in this NHQR, quality of care is considerably and consistently worse for patients with no insurance compared with patients who have private insurance. In addition, nearly two-thirds of patients who are unable to get or delayed in getting needed care report a reason related to cost or insurance. Quality improvement will be impeded as long as more than 46 million Americans are uninsured and face barriers to quality health care.[7]

The **Office of Health Reform** (http://healthreform.gov) leads and coordinates the Federal Government's comprehensive effort to improve health care so that it is high quality, affordable, accessible, and sustainable. The Office envisions reform that will reduce long-term growth in health care costs for businesses and government; protect families from bankruptcy or debt because of health care costs; guarantee choice of doctors and health plans; invest in prevention and wellness; improve patient safety and quality of care; ensure affordable, quality health coverage for all Americans; maintain coverage when individuals change or lose their job; and end barriers to coverage for people with preexisting medical conditions.[8] Achieving these goals could dramatically reduce the number of uninsured Americans and improve health care quality.

Empower Providers with Health Information Technology and Training

HIT needs to support quality improvement. Providers need reliable information about their performance to guide improvement activities. Realistically, HIT infrastructure is needed to ensure that relevant data are collected regularly, systematically, and unobtrusively while protecting patient privacy and confidentiality. Patients, including individuals with limited English proficiency or disabilities, need to have meaningful access to their health records to ensure accuracy and completeness. Systems need to generate information that can be understood by end users and that are interoperable across different institutions' data platforms, policies, and procedures.[9] In addition, information systems are necessary but insufficient for ensuring high-quality health care.[10]

Quality improvement typically requires examining patterns of care across panels of patients rather than one patient at a time. Unfortunately, information systems often are not designed to collect data to support quality improvement as the primary purpose. Retrofitting legacy health information systems to capture data on quality measures is often labor intensive. Also, many benefits of improved information technologies require systems that go beyond simple automated recordkeeping.[11] Ideally, performance measures should be calculated automatically from health records in a format that can be easily shared and compared across all providers involved with a patient's care.

The **American Recovery and Reinvestment Act** (ARRA) provides reimbursement incentives for providers to adopt electronic health records and to achieve meaningful use of them. CMS and the Office of the National Coordinator are currently working on the operational definition of meaningful use. The conceptual framework recognizes that meaningful use may begin with data capture and sharing but must progress to decision support of care processes and ultimately yield improvements in health outcomes.

Training is also critical. Improving quality is a "team sport." TeamSTEPPS™ (Team Strategies and Tools to Enhance Performance and Patient Safety, http://teamstepps.ahrq.gov) is an evidence-based teamwork system aimed at optimizing patient outcomes by improving health professionals' communication and teamwork skills. It includes a comprehensive set of ready-to-use materials and a training curriculum to integrate teamwork principles into any health care system. In collaboration with AHRQ, the Department of Defense developed TeamSTEPPS and has built a national training and support network called the National Implementation of TeamSTEPPS Project. This network is currently conducting training sessions throughout the country.

AHRQ is also supporting training of multidisciplinary hospital teams to address HAIs. **The Keystone ICU Project** helped 108 intensive care units in Michigan reduce rates of bloodstream infections associated with central venous catheters. AHRQ is currently working to develop tools to teach additional hospitals how to reduce these types of complications.

Think Cultural Health (http://www.ThinkCulturalHealth.org), developed by the Office of Minority Health (OMH), offers a suite of cultural competency training programs, including *A Physician's Practical Guide to Culturally Competent Care, Culturally Competent Nursing Care,* and the *Health Care Language Services Implementation Guide*. These free online programs allow busy health professionals to earn continuing education credits in an atmosphere of their choosing and at their own pace. Institutions can follow a small group format that allows a team to train, discuss, and plan together based on the organization's needs and experiences. In addition to continuing education, the Web site houses up-to-date information on cultural competency legislation, health disparities, and health care for racial and ethnic minorities.

Establish and Sustain Partnerships to Lead Change

Partnerships need to build health care quality and cost information systems nationwide. Quality measures often provide narrow views of system performance rather than the comprehensive picture needed to optimize care. The Quality Alliance Steering Committee (http://www.healthqualityalliance.org) is a partnership of quality and health care leaders that is building an infrastructure for gathering and reporting consistent, effective, and efficient information on health care quality and costs. Through its High-Value Health Care Project, the committee is devising solutions that will allow efficient aggregation and integration of health care data from public and private sectors, developing measures of costs and efficiency, and supporting consistent collection of standardized race and ethnicity identifiers that will advance understanding of equity in health care quality.

Partnerships are needed to effect change and do the actual work of making improvements. The National Priorities Partnership (http://www.nationalpriorities partner ship.org) is a collaborative effort of key public and private health care stakeholders. The partners have agreed on a core set of national health care priorities and goals that they will work together to achieve. These priorities include patient and family engagement, population health, safety, care coordination, palliative and end-of-life care, and overuse.

The National Partnership for Action (NPA) To End Health Disparities (http://minorityhealth.hhs.gov/npa), launched by OMH, is a multifaceted effort to mobilize and connect individuals and organizations across the country to create a Nation free of health disparities, with quality health outcomes for all people. The NPA is composed of three components: (1) National Plan for Action; (2) 10 Regional Blueprints aligned with the National Plan for Action that include strategies and actions most pertinent to communities in each region; and (3) targeted initiatives that will be undertaken by partners across the public and private sectors in support of the NPA.

An example of an NPA initiative is the National Business Group on Health Racial and Ethnic Health Disparities Advisory Board. This advisory board facilitates alliances between business, medicine, and public health organizations to improve the quality of health care for racial and ethnic minority populations while promoting beneficiary health and employee productivity. Products include issue briefs on topics such as why companies are making health disparities their business and how health plans view health disparities. The board holds several Web conferences featuring best practices by a wide range of employers.

Conclusion

Quality improvement requires measurement and reporting, but these are not the ultimate goals. The fundamental purpose of quality improvement in health care is to make patients' and families' lives better. The NHQR concentrates on tracking health care quality at the national level, but the statistics reported in the NHQR and NHDR reflect the aggregated everyday experiences of patients and their providers across the Nation. It makes a difference in people's lives when breast cancer is diagnosed early with timely mammography; when a patient suffering from a heart attack is given the correct lifesaving treatment in a timely fashion; when medications are correctly administered; and when doctors listen to their patients and their families, show them respect, and answer their questions.

With the publication of this seventh NHQR, AHRQ stands ready to contribute to efforts that encourage and support the development of national, State, Tribal, and "neighborhood" solutions using national data and benchmarks in quality. This chapter documents some areas where important progress has been achieved in improving patients' quality of life, as well as many areas where much more should be done. It also points to important opportunities that still exist.

We need to accelerate the pace of quality improvement, especially related to patient safety. Barriers to quality health care, such as uninsurance, need to be overcome. The success of CMS reporting initiatives may serve as a guide, but more work is needed to improve, standardize, and coordinate quality measurement. Information on quality then needs to be shared with partners who have the skills and commitment to change health care. Building on data in the NHQR, NHDR, and the State Snapshots, we believe that policymakers can design and target strategies and clinical interventions to ensure that patients receive the highest quality care that makes their lives better.

REFERENCES

[1] Institute of Medicine. Crossing the quality chasm: a new health system for the 21st century. *Washington, DC*: National Academies Press; 2001.

[2] Keehan, S; Sisko, A; Truffer, C. et al. Health spending projections through 2017: the Baby-Boom generation is coming to Medicare. *Health Aff (Millwood)* 2008 Mar-Apr, 27(2), w145-55.

[3] Kohn, L; Corrigan, J; Donaldson, M. eds. To err is human: building a safer health system. Washington, DC: Institute of Medicine, *Committee on Quality of Health Care in America*; 2000.

[4] Aspden, P; Corrigan, J; Wolcott, J. et al. *Patient safety: achieving a new standard of care*. Washington, DC: Institute of Medicine, Committee on Data Standards for Patient Safety; 2004.

[5] Adams, K; Corrigan, J. *Priority areas for national action: transforming health care quality*. Washington, DC: Institute of Medicine, Committee on Identifying Priority Areas for Quality Improvement, Board of Healthcare Services; 2003.

[6] National Priorities Partnership. *National priorities and goals: aligning our efforts to transform America's healthcare*. Washington, DC: National Quality Forum; 2008.

[7] DeNavas-Walt, C; Proctor, B; Smith, JC. Income, poverty, and health insurance coverage in the United States: 2008. Washington, DC: U.S. Department of Commerce, Census Bureau, Economics and Statistics Administration; 2009. No. P60-236. Available at: www.census.gov/prod/2009pubs/p60-236.pdf. Accessed on October 8, 2009.
[8] Sebelius, K. Statement on health reform in the 21st century before Committee on Ways and Means. Washington, DC: U.S. House of Representatives; May 6, 2009. Available at: http://waysandmeans.house.gov/hearings.asp?formmode=view&id=7734.
[9] Clancy, CM; Anderson, KM; White, PJ. Investing in health information infrastructure: can it help achieve health reform? *Health Aff (Millwood)* 2009 Mar-Apr, 28(2), 478-82.
[10]Linder, JA; Ma, J; Bates, DW. et al. Electronic health record use and the quality of ambulatory care in the United States. *Arch Intern Med,* 2007 Jul 9, 167(13), 1400-5.
[11]Amarasingham, R; Plantinga, L; Diener-West, M. et al. Clinical information technologies and inpatient outcomes: a multiple hospital study. *Arch Intern Med* 2009 Jan 26, 169(2), 108-14.

1. Introduction and Methods

In 1999, Congress directed the Agency for Healthcare Research and Quality (AHRQ) to produce an annual report, starting in 2003, on health care quality in the United States (42 U.S.C. 299b-2(b)(2)). AHRQ, with support from the Department of Health and Human Services and private-sector partners, has designed and produced the National Healthcare Quality Report (NHQR) to respond to this legislative mandate.

This is the seventh annual report on the state of health care quality nationally. Similar to the previous six reports, it is designed to summarize data across a wide range of patient needs, including staying healthy, getting better, living with chronic illness and disability, and coping with the end of life. The main purpose of the report is to show readers the extent to which care in the United States is delivered in an effective, safe, timely, patient-centered, and efficient manner.

The first NHQR was a comprehensive national overview of the quality of health care that the general U.S. population received. The 2004 NHQR initiated a second critical goal of the report series: tracking the Nation's quality improvement progress. The 2005 NHQR introduced a set of core measures and a variety of new composite measures. The 2006 NHQR continued to improve data, measures, and methods, adding databases and measures and refining methods for quantifying and tracking changes in health care. The 2007 NHQR launched a new chapter on health care efficiency. The 2008 NHQR included an expanded chapter on patient safety.

This chapter summarizes the methodological approaches AHRQ has taken in producing the 2009 NHQR. Material that is new in this year's report includes sections on:

- Health care-associated infections.
- Patient safety culture in hospitals.
- Pain management among home health care and hospice patients.
- Care coordination.

- Potentially avoidable hospitalizations among home health care and nursing home patients.
- Efficiency of care for congestive heart failure.
- Reduction of unnecessary costs.

As in previous years, the 2009 NHQR was written by AHRQ staff, with the support and guidance of AHRQ's National Advisory Council and the Interagency Work Group for the NHQR.

How This Chapter Is Organized

The basic structure of the report consists of the following:

- **Highlights** summarizes key themes and highlights from the 2008 report.
- **Section 1: Introduction and Methods** documents the organization, data sources, and methods used in the 2009 report and describes major changes from previous reports.
- **Section 2: Effectiveness** examines the quality of health care in the general U.S. population. This year, this chapter has been reorganized around eight clinical areas (cancer, diabetes, end stage renal disease, heart disease, HIV and AIDS, maternal and child health, mental health and substance abuse, and respiratory diseases) and three types of health care services that typically cut across clinical conditions (lifestyle modification, functional status preservation and rehabilitation, and supportive and palliative care). Measures of the quality of health care used in this chapter are identical to measures used in the National Healthcare Disparities Report (NHDR) except when data to examine disparities are unavailable for inclusion in the NHDR.
- **Section 3: Patient Safety** tracks measures of patient safety, including health care-associated infections, postoperative complications, other complications of hospital care, and complications of medications. A new section this year focuses on patient safety culture in hospitals and indicates the extent to which hospital staff incorporate patient safety principles and practices into their work.
- **Section 4: Timeliness** examines the delivery of time-sensitive clinical care and patient perceptions of the timeliness and accessibility of their care.
- **Section 5: Patient Centeredness** tracks patients' experiences with care in an office or clinic and satisfaction with communication during a hospital stay in order to incorporate the patient's experience and perspective into the report. This year's chapter also includes a new section on care coordination.
- **Section 6: Efficiency** presents a conceptual view and an expanded set of analyses of this dimension of health care performance. Efficiency was first introduced in the 2007 NHQR.

Measure Set for the NHQR and NHDR

The NHQR and NHDR track a broad array of health care measures and have added measures each year. In this chapter, we begin the process of trimming the measure set by retiring some measures that have attained high levels of overall performance. As in previous years, the 2009 reports focus on a subset of core report measures. In addition, composite measures are included to provide readers with a summary picture of some aspect of health care by combining information from multiple component measures.

Retired Measures

Previous NHQRs have demonstrated that most measures of health care quality tend to improve. Since the first NHQR, significant improvements in a number of measures of quality of care have occurred. U.S. health care providers have achieved overall performance levels exceeding 95% on five measures tracked in past NHQRs.

The measures that have achieved 95% performance are:

- Adults with diabetes who had their blood cholesterol checked.
- Hospital patients with heart attack who received aspirin within 24 hours of admission.
- Hospital patients with heart attack who were prescribed aspirin at discharge.
- Hospital patients with heart attack who were prescribed a beta blocker at discharge.
- Smokers with heart attack who received smoking cessation counseling while hospitalized.

The success of these measures limits their utility for tracking improvement over time. Because these measures cannot improve further to a significant degree, including them in the measure set creates a ceiling effect that may distort quantification of rate of change over time. Hence, we have retired these measures from our measure set for tracking purposes. However, we will continue to gather data on them and will add them back if their performance falls below 95%.

Core Measures

This 2009 NHQR continues to focus on a consistent subset of measures, the "core" measures, which includes the most important and scientifically supported measures in the full NHQR measure set. In 2005, the Interagency Work Group selected the core measures from the full measure sets and findings based on the measures presented each year. In addition, "noncore" measures are included in summary statistics and may be presented to complement core measures in key areas. For some topics, the NHQR uses alternating sets of core measures. These measures, are listed in Table 1.1. All alternating core measures are included in analyses of rate change.

All core measures fall into two categories: process measures, which track receipt of medical services; and outcome measures, which in part reflect the results of medical care. Both types of measures are not reported for all conditions due to data limitations. For example, data on HIV care are suboptimal; hence, no HIV process measures are included as core measures. In addition, not all core measures are included in trending analysis, because 2 or more years of data are not always available. Ideally, process measures and the outcome measures they could affect would be tracked in tandem. However, data to support such process-outcome measurement pairs are not typically available. Related process and outcome core measures in the 2009 NHQR measure set are listed in Table 1.2. Other core measures are listed in Table 1.3.

Composite Measures

In some cases, measures can be combined to form a single composite measure of health care quality. A composite measure summarizes care that is represented by individual measures that are often related in some way, such as components of care for a particular disease or illness. Policymakers and others have voiced their support for composite measures because they can be used to facilitate understanding of information from many individual measures. The effort to develop new composites is ongoing and, in 2006, a number of composite measures were added.[V] The complete list of composite measures is shown in Table 1.4.

Table 1.1. Alternating Core Measures

Presented in 2008 NHQR and NHDR*	Presented in 2009 NHQR and NHDR
Colorectal cancer screening	Breast cancer screening (mammography)
Colorectal cancer mortality	Breast cancer mortality
Colorectal cancer diagnosis at advanced stage	Breast cancer diagnosis at advanced stage
Children who had a vision check	Children who had a dental visit

* The measures listed in this column will be presented again in the 2010 reports.

Composite measures in the NHQR are created in a variety of different ways. The appropriateness model is sometimes referred to as the "all-or-none" approach because it is calculated based on the number of patients who received all of the services they needed. One example of this model is the diabetes composite, in which a patient who receives only one or two of the three services would not be counted as having received all recommended care.

The opportunities model assumes that each patient needs and has the opportunity to receive one or more processes of care, but not all patients need the same care. Composite measures that use this model summarize the proportion of appropriate care that is delivered. The denominator for an opportunities model composite is the sum of opportunities to receive appropriate care across a panel of process measures. The numerator is the sum of the components of appropriate care that are actually delivered. The composite measure of recommended hospital care for heart failure is an example where this model is applied. The total number of patients who receive treatments represented by individual components of the composite measure (e.g., evaluation of left ventricular ejection fraction and ACE inhibitor or ARB among patients with left ventricular systolic dysfunction) is divided by the sum of all of these opportunities to receive appropriate care.

Measures from the CAHPS® (Consumer Assessment of Healthcare Providers and Systems) surveys have their own method for computing composite measures that has been in use for many years. These composite measures average individual components of patient experiences of care. They are typically presented as the proportion of respondents who reported that providers sometimes or never, usually, or always performed well.

Table 1.2. Related Core Process and Outcome Measures (Measures without New Data in Italics)

Section	Process measures	Outcome measures
Effectiveness: Cancer	• Women age 40 and over who reported they had a ammogram within the past 2 years	• Rate of advanced stage breast cancer per 100,000 women age 40 and over • Breast cancer deaths per 100,000 women
Effectiveness: Diabetes	• Adults age 40 and over with diagnosed diabetes who received all three recommen-ded services for diabetes in the calendar year (hemoglobin A1c measurement, dilated eye examination, and foot examination	• *Hospital admissions for lower extremity amputation per 1,000 population age 18 and over with diabetes*
Effectiveness: Maternal and Child Health	• *Women who completed a pregnancy in the last 12 months who first received prenatal care in the first trimester* • Children ages 19-35 months who received all recommended vaccines • Children ages 2-17 with a dental visit in the calendar year • Children ages 2-17 for whom a health provider gave advice about physical activity • Children ages 2-17 for whom a health provider gave advice about healthy eating	• *Infant deaths per 1,000 live births, birth weight <1,500 grams*
Effectiveness: Mental Health and Substance Abuse	• Adults with a major depressive episode in the past year who received treatment for depression • People age 12 and over who needed treatment for illicit drug use or an alcohol problem and who received such treatment at a specialty facility in the last 12 months	• Suicide deaths per 100,000 population
Effectiveness: Supportive and Palliative Care	• Long-stay nursing home residents with physical restraints	• High-risk long-stay nursing home residents with pressure sores • Short-stay nursing home residents with pressure sores • Adult home health care patients with shortness of breath

Table 1.3. Other Core Process and Outcome Measures

Section	Process measures	Outcome measures
Effectiveness: End Stage Renal Disease	• Dialysis patients who were registered on a waiting list for transplantation	• Adult hemodialysis patients with adequate dialysis (urea reduction ratio 65% or greater)
Effectiveness: Heart Disease	• Hospital patients with heart attack and left ventricular systolic dysfunction who received angiotensin-converting enzyme (ACE) inhibitor or angiotensin receptor blocker (ARB) • Hospital patients with heart failure who received recommended hospital care (evaluation of left ventricular ejection fraction and ACE inhibitor or ARB prescription at discharge, if indicated, for left ventricular systolic dysfunction)	• Deaths per 1,000 adult hospital admissions with heart attack
Effectiveness: HIV and AIDS	(HIV process measures tracked in the NHQR are noncore.)	• New AIDS cases per 100,000 population age 13 and over
Effectiveness: Respiratory Diseases	• Adults age 65 and over who ever received pneumococcal vaccination • Hospital patients with pneumonia who received recommended hospital care (blood culture collected before first antibiotic dose, initial antibiotic dose within 6 hours of hospital arrival and consistent with current recommendations, and influenza and pneumococcal screening or vaccination) • People with current asthma who are now taking preventive medicine daily or almost daily	• Patients with tuberculosis who completed a curative course of treatment within 1 year of initiation of treatment
Effectiveness: Lifestyle Modification	• Adult current smokers with a checkup in the last 12 months who received advice to quit smoking • Adults with obesity who ever received advice from a health provider to exercise more	• (No outcomes of lifestyle modification are currently tracked in the NHQR.)

Table 1.3. (Continued)

Section	Process measures	Outcome measures
Effectiveness: Functional Status Preservation and Rehabilitation	• Older women who ever reported being screened for osteoporosis	• Adult home health care patients whose ability to walk or move around improved • Nursing home residents whose need for help with daily activities increased
Patient Safety	• Adult surgery patients who received appropriate timing of antibiotics • Adults age 65 and over who received potentially inappropriate prescription medications	• Adult surgery patients with postoperative complications (postoperative pneumonia or venous thromboembolic event) • Bloodstream infections or mechanical adverse events associated with central venous catheter placement
Timeliness		• Adults who needed care right away for an illness, injury, or condition in the last 12 months who did not get care as soon as wanted • Emergency department visits in which patients left without being seen
Patient Centeredness	• Adult ambulatory patients who reported poor communication with health providers • Children with ambulatory visits whose parents reported poor communication with health providers	

Composite measures that relate to rates of complications of hospital care are postoperative complications and complications of central venous catheters. For these complication rate composites, an additive model is used that sums individual complication rates. Thus, for these composites, the numerator is the sum of individual complications and the denominator is the number of patients at risk for these complications. The composite rates are presented as the overall rate of complications. The postoperative complications composite is a good example of this type of composite measure: If 50 patients had a total of 15 complications among them (regardless of their distribution), the composite score would be 30%.

Table 1.4. Composite Measures in the 2009 NHQR and NHDR

Composite measure	Individual measures forming composite	Model
Receipt of three recommended diabetes services	• Adults age 40 and over with diagnosed diabetes who had a hemoglobin A1c measurement in the calendar year • Adults age 40 and over with diagnosed diabetes who had a dilated eye examination in the calendar year • Adults age 40 and over with diagnosed diabetes who had a foot examination in the calendar year	Appropriateness
Childhood Immunization[VI]	• Children ages 19-35 months who received 4 doses of diphtheria-tetanus-acellular pertussis vaccine • Children ages 19-35 months who received 3 doses of polio vaccine • Children ages 19-35 months who received 1 dose of measles-mumps-rubella vaccine • Children ages 19-35 months who received 3 doses of *Haemophilus influenzae* type B vaccine • Children ages 19-35 months who received 3 doses of hepatitis B vaccine	Appropriateness
Recommended hospital care for heart failure	• Hospital patients with heart failure who received an evaluation of left ventricular ejection fraction • Hospital patients with heart failure and left ventricular systolic dysfunction who were prescribed ACE inhibitor or ARB at discharge	Opportunities
Recommended hospital care for pneumonia	• Hospital patients with pneumonia who had blood cultures collected before antibiotics were administered • Hospital patients with pneumonia who received the initial antibiotic dose within 6 hours of hospital arrival • Hospital patients with pneumonia who received the initial antibiotic consistent with current recommendations • Hospital patients with pneumonia who received influenza screening or vaccination • Hospital patients with pneumonia who received pneumococcal screening or vaccination	Opportunities
Timing of antibiotics to prevent postoperative wound infection	• Adult surgery patients who received prophylactic antibiotics within 1 hour prior to surgical incision • Adult surgery patients who had prophylactic antibiotics discontinued within 24 hours after surgery end time	Opportunities

Table 1.4. (Continued)

Composite measure	Individual measures forming composite	Model
Patients' experience of care	• Adult ambulatory patients whose providers sometimes or never listened carefully to them • Adult ambulatory patients whose providers sometimes or never explained things in a way they could understand • Adult ambulatory patients whose providers sometimes or never showed respect for what they had to say • Adult ambulatory patients whose providers sometimes or never spent enough time with them • Children with ambulatory visits whose parents report that their child's providers sometimes or never listened carefully to them • Children with ambulatory visits whose parents report that their child's providers sometimes or never explained things in a way they could understand • Children with ambulatory visits whose parents report that their child's providers sometimes or never showed respect for what they had to say • Children with ambulatory visits whose parents report that their child's providers sometimes or never spent enough time with them	CAHPS®
Postoperative complications	• Adult surgery patients with postoperative pneumonia events	Additive
	• Adult surgery patients with postoperative venous thromboembolic events	
Complications of central venous catheters	• Bloodstream infections among central venous catheter placements • Mechanical adverse events per 1,000 central venous catheter placements	Additive

Presentation

As in past reports, the NHQR and its companion NHDR continue to be formatted as chartbooks. Each section in the 2009 report begins with a description of the importance of the section's topic in a standardized format. After introductory text, charts and accompanying findings highlight a small number of measures relevant to the topic. Sometimes these charts show contrasts by age, when age data are available and relevant.

Almost all core measures and composite measures have multiple years of data, so figures typically illustrate trends over time. Figures include a notation about the denominator, either the reference population for population-based measures or the unit of analysis for measures based on services or events from provider- or establishment-based data collection efforts.

New themes emphasized in this chapter include exploring the effects of health insurance on quality of care and examining State variation in processes and outcomes together. The NHDR has identified insurance as an important determinant of disparities in health care. To systematically identify the relationship between insurance and quality of care, when possible, findings in the NHQR show measures of quality of care for individuals with different types of insurance. For those under age 65, individuals with any private insurance, public insurance only, and no insurance are typically compared. For those age 65 and over, individuals with Medicare and private insurance, Medicare and other public insurance, and Medicare only are typically compared.

Previous NHQRs have shown that wide variation exists across States in processes and outcomes of health care. This year, the NHQR introduces a new type of State variation map. Rather than focus on a single process or outcome measure, these maps identify States that perform poorly on both a process measure and a related outcome measure. These maps do not imply causality; improvements in processes of care typically affect outcomes some time in the future. Rather, these maps are intended to help identify those States that may have the greatest motivation to improve performance in this area. These maps generally focus on States in the worst performing quartile of process and outcome measures.

In addition, to place findings in the context of other Federal reporting initiatives, this chapter indicates where NHQR measures are also included in Healthy People 2010. Note that the Healthy People 2010 targets represented in the report figures, where applicable, reflect target values that were current when the reports were being prepared. Targets may be revised as new information becomes available. Therefore, the targets shown on the figures may differ from those in past reports or subsequent revisions. Also, Healthy People 2010 targets are only referenced in relation to the total population, not particular age groups. In addition, the data source for estimates reported here must be the same as the Healthy People 2010 data source in order for comparisons to be made.

Databases

Table 1.5 lists the databases used in the 2009 reports.

Table 1.5. Databases Used in the 2009 Reports (new data sources in italics)

Survey data collected from populations
• AHRQ, Medical Expenditure Panel Survey (MEPS), 2000-2006
• Centers for Disease Control and Prevention (CDC), Behavioral Risk Factor Surveillance System (BRFSS), 2003-2006
• CDC-National Center for Health Statistics (NCHS), National Health and Nutrition Examination Survey (NHANES), 1999-2006
• CDC-NCHS, National Health Interview Survey (NHIS), 1998-2007
• CDC-NCHS and National Center for Immunization and Respiratory Diseases, National Immunization Survey (NIS), 2000-2007
• Centers for Medicare & Medicaid Services (CMS), Medicare Current Beneficiary Survey (MCBS), 1998-2004
• Health Resources and Services Administration (HRSA) and CDC-NCHS, National Survey of Children With Special Health Care Needs (NSCSHCN), 2005-2006
• *Massachusetts Health Quality Partners (MHQP), Patient Experience Survey, 2007*
• National Hospice and Palliative Care Organization, Family Evaluation of Hospice Care, 2005-2008

Table 1.5. (Continued)
Survey data collected from populations
• Substance Abuse and Mental Health Services Administration (SAMHSA), National Survey on Drug Use and Health (NSDUH), 2002-2007
• U.S. Census Bureau, American Community Survey, 2007
Data collected from samples of health care facilities and providers
• *AHRQ, Hospital Survey on Patient Safety Culture, 2008*
• American Cancer Society and American College of Surgeons, National Cancer Data Base (NCDB), 2000-2006
• CDC-NCHS, National Ambulatory Medical Care Survey (NAMCS), 1997-2007
• *CDC-NCHS, National Home and Hospice Care Survey, 2007*
• CDC-NCHS, National Hospital Ambulatory Medical Care Survey-Emergency Department (NHAMCS-ED), 1997-2007
• CDC-NCHS, National Hospital Ambulatory Medical Care Survey-Outpatient Department (NHAMCS-OPD), 1997-2007
• CDC-NCHS, National Hospital Discharge Survey (NHDS), 1998-2006
• CMS, End Stage Renal Disease Clinical Performance Measures Project (ESRD CPMP), 2002-2007
Data extracted from data systems of health care organizations
• *AHRQ, Healthcare Cost and Utilization Project (HCUP), Nationwide Emergency Department Sample (NEDS), 2005*
• AHRQ, HCUP, Nationwide Inpatient Sample (NIS), 2004-2006, and State Inpatient Databases (SID), a 2006
• CMS, Home Health Outcomes and Assessment Information Set (OASIS), 2002-2008
• CMS, Hospital Compare, 2008
• *CMS, Medicare National Claims History, 2000-2006*
• CMS, Medicare Patient Safety Monitoring System (MPSMS), 2004-2007
• CMS, Nursing Home Minimum Data Set (MDS), 2000-2008
• CMS, Quality Improvement Organization (QIO) program, Hospital Quality Alliance (HQA) measures, 2002-2007
• HIV Research Network (HIVRN) data, 2004-2006
• Indian Health Service, National Patient Information Reporting System (NPIRS), 2003-2006
• National Committee for Quality Assurance, Health Plan Employer Data and Information Set (HEDIS®), 2001-2005
• National Institutes of Health (NIH), United States Renal Data System (USRDS), 2000-2005
• SAMHSA, Treatment Episode Data Set (TEDS), 2002-2005
Data from surveillance and vital statistics systems
• CDC-National Center for HIV, Viral Hepatitis, STD, and TB Prevention, HIV/AIDS Reporting System, 2000-2007
• CDC-National Center for HIV, STD, and TB Prevention, TB Surveillance System, 2000-2005
• CDC-National Program of Cancer Registries (NPCR), 2000-2004
• CDC-NCHS, National Vital Statistics System (NVSS), 1999-2006
• NIH-National Cancer Institute, Surveillance, Epidemiology, and End Results (SEER) program, 2000-2006

[a] Not all States participate in HCUP. For details, see HCUP entry in Appendix A, Data Sources.

Note: Measures from the American Community Survey are used only in the NHDR. For details on these surveys, refer to Chapter 1, Introduction and Methods, in the 2009 NHDR.

Analyses

This section summarizes the methodologies behind the analyses shown in the report. Unless otherwise specified, only findings that meet our criteria for significance are discussed in the text of this chapter.

For all measures, analyses are conducted to assess change over time. For individual measures, the average annual rate of change is calculated between the earliest and the most recent estimates within a specified date range. Consistent with *Health, United States*, a formula that produces the geometric rate of change is used for this calculation for each measure.[VII] This geometric rate of change assumes the same rate of change each year between the two time periods. For each measure discussed in the reports, two criteria are then applied to determine whether a meaningful trend exists:

- First, the difference between the oldest and most recent estimates must be statistically significant with alpha≤0.05 on a two-tailed test.
- Second, the average annual rate of change must be at least 1% per year when the measure is framed either positively as a favorable outcome or negatively as an adverse outcome.

For example, assume a favorable outcome, receipt of a needed service, increased from 90% to 94% over a 5-year period. To assess meaningfulness, statistical significance of this difference would first be assessed using a two-tailed test. If significant with alpha≤0.05, the average annual rate of change would then be calculated using the geometric rate of change formula. In this case, $[(94/90)^{1/5}-1]$ x100 yields an average annual rate of change of 0.9% per year, less than our threshold of 1% per year. The measure is then converted into an adverse outcome, lack of receipt of a needed service, which decreased from 10% to 6% over the time period. Applying the geometric rate of change formula, $[(6/10)^{1/5}-1]$ x100, yields an average annual rate of change of -9.7% per year. Because this rate of change with the measure framed negatively as an adverse outcome exceeds our 1% threshold, we consider this change to be meaningful.

In addition, many measures are tracked for different groups defined by age or insurance status, and comparisons among groups are made. In general, the largest groups are used as the standard reference groups; unless specified, this would typically be individuals ages 18-44 for age contrasts and individuals with private health insurance for insurance contrasts. Two criteria are applied to determine whether the difference between two groups is meaningful:

- First, the difference between the two groups must be statistically significant with alpha≤0.05 on a two-tailed test.
- Second, the relative difference between the comparison group and the reference group must be at least 10% when the measure is framed either positively as a favorable outcome or negatively as an adverse outcome.

In the Highlights chapter, we also summarize rates of change over time across broad panels of measures. This process is more complicated because data on all measures are not collected each year. Therefore, specifying the optimal time period for analysis without excluding large numbers of measures has been a challenge. Specific issues include:

- Changes in the measure set over time.
- Changes in the data source over time.
- Lack of availability of data for particular data years.
- Recalculation of prior years' data.

Changes in the measure set may result from the deletion of measures due to lack of availability of new data or a determination by the NHQR's Interagency Work Group that a measure no longer meets its criteria for inclusion. Changes also result from the addition of a measure. For example, this chapter includes a core measure for daily use of preventive medicine for current asthma. This measure was added in 2008 and uses data from AHRQ's Medical Expenditure Panel Survey (MEPS). Data for this measure were first collected in 2003. The latest MEPS data year available for this NHQR was 2006. Therefore, for this measure data were only available for 4 years: 2003, 2004, 2005, and 2006. A 5-year or longer period might be available for other measures.

For this and other reasons (e.g., variability of collection schedules among the different data sources used by the NHQR), if a strict time-interval criterion for trend analysis were used (e.g., only the 2000 and 2006 data years), a large number of measures would be excluded. The approach taken for this year's report favors inclusion of as many measures as possible over a strict application of a minimum number of data points or time interval.

For this year's summary trend analyses, for each measure, we obtain all available data points between the year 2000 and the current data year. Linear regression is applied to these data and the slope of the regression line is used as the estimate of change over time.[VIII] Across different panels of measures, these estimates are then summarized as means and medians.

One other methodological issue should be noted. Composite measures are included in the core measure category. To avoid duplication of estimates within the other categories, composite measures are not included in other categories where estimates from their component measures are used. For example, the diabetes composite measure (which includes HbA1c measurement, eye exam, and foot exam) contributes to the overall rate for the core measures group but not to the diabetes group rate, which uses the estimates from the three noncore component measures.

Various words and phrases might be used to refer to a change, depending on the specific measure being discussed. For example, "more likely to," "significantly below," "decreased," "had the highest rate," "change," "improvement," "statistically higher," and "less likely to" all refer to changes that meet the two criteria listed above. Although the explicit use of the term "statistically significant" is warranted in some cases, imposing its use in every sentence where a change is discussed would be overly cumbersome. Also, not every significant change among data years or populations is noted. Therefore, no conclusions should be drawn if a numeric difference in a figure is not referenced in the corresponding text or bullet.

Due to the methodological changes discussed here, changes to estimates for data from prior years, and changes to the measure set, it is not appropriate to compare the rates of change for measure groups discussed in this year's report with those from prior years.

Finally, this chapter conforms to the Government Printing Office Style Manual. In some cases, terms or spelling may vary to reflect an original data source or an agency or program name. For example, "health care" usually appears as two words but may appear as one word in an agency name, such as the Agency for Healthcare Research and Quality. These minor variations in spelling and usage do not alter the meaning or intent of the data and are purely cosmetic in nature.

2. Effectiveness

As better understanding of health and sickness has led to superior ways of preventing, diagnosing, and treating diseases, the health of most Americans has improved dramatically. However, ample evidence indicates that some Americans do not receive the full benefits of high-quality care. As noted in Chapter 1, Introduction and Methods, this year's findings include an assessment of the effects of health insurance on quality of care.

When possible, findings in this chapter show measures of effectiveness of care for individuals with different types of insurance. For those under age 65, individuals with any private insurance, public insurance only, and no insurance are typically compared. For those age 65 and over, individuals with Medicare and private insurance, Medicare and other public insurance, and Medicare only are typically compared. Differences in care according to insurance status may reflect the direct impact of insurance coverage on access to and quality of services. But other factors may play a part, such as differences in personal decisions, social norms, and communication styles across groups with differing levels of insurance.

In addition, this year's sections on effectiveness of care have been reorganized. This chapter is organized around eight clinical areas (cancer, diabetes, end stage renal disease, heart disease, HIV and AIDS, maternal and child health, mental health and substance abuse, and respiratory diseases) and three types of health care services that typically cut across clinical conditions (lifestyle modification, functional status preservation and rehabilitation, and supportive and palliative care). The 11 sections of this chapter highlight a small number of core measures.

In this chapter, process measures are organized into several categories related to the patient's need for preventive care, treatment of acute illness, and chronic disease management. These are derived from the original Institute of Medicine categories: staying healthy, getting better, living with illness or disability, and coping with the end of life. There is sizable overlap among these categories, and some measures may be considered to belong in more than one category. Outcome measures are organized separately because prevention, treatment, and management can all play important roles in affecting outcomes.

Prevention

Caring for healthy people is an important component of health care. Educating people about health and promoting healthy behaviors can help postpone or avoid illness and disease. In addition, detecting health problems at an early stage increases the chances of effectively treating them, often reducing suffering and costs.

Treatment

Even when preventive care is ideally implemented, it cannot entirely avert the need for acute care. Delivering optimal treatments for acute illness can help reduce the consequences of illness and promote the best recovery possible.

Section	Measure
Prevention	
Cancer	Breast cancer screening (mammography)
Maternal and child health	Recommended immunization of young children
Maternal and child health	Dental visits for children
Maternal and child health	Weight monitoring of overweight children*
Maternal and child health	Counseling for children about physical activity
Maternal and child health	Counseling for children about healthy eating
Respiratory diseases	Pneumococcal vaccination
Lifestyle modification	Counseling smokers to quit smoking
Lifestyle modification	Counseling obese adults about overweight*
Lifestyle modification	Counseling obese adults about exercise
Functional status preservation and rehabilitation	Osteoporosis screening in women
Treatment	
Cancer	Women with clinical Stage I-IIb breast cancer who received axillary node dissection or sentinel lymph node biopsy*
Cancer	Women treated with breast-conserving surgery who received radiation therapy*
Heart disease	Angiotensin-converting enzyme inhibitor or angiotensin receptor blocker for heart attack
Heart disease	Recommended care for heart failure
Mental health and substance abuse	Treatment for depression
Mental health and substance abuse	Treatment for illicit drug use or alcohol problem
Mental health and substance abuse	Completion of substance abuse treatment*
Respiratory diseases	Recommended care for pneumonia
Management	
Diabetes	Recommended diabetes services
End stage renal disease	Registration for transplantation
HIV and AIDS	*Pneumocystis* pneumonia and *Mycobacterium avium* complex prophylaxis*
Respiratory diseases	Daily asthma medication
Supportive and palliative care	Use of physical restraints on long-stay nursing home residents
Supportive and palliative care	Referral to hospice at the right time*
Supportive and palliative care	Receipt of right amount of pain medicine by hospice patients*
Outcome	
Cancer	Breast cancer first diagnosed at advanced stage
Cancer	Breast cancer deaths
Diabetes	Control of hemoglobin A1c, cholesterol, and blood pressure*
End stage renal disease	Adequate hemodialysis
Heart disease	Inpatient deaths following heart attack
HIV and AIDS	New AIDS cases
HIV and AIDS	HIV infection deaths*
Maternal and child health	Obstetric trauma*

Table. (Continued)	
Section	**Measure**
Mental health and substance abuse	Suicide deaths
Respiratory diseases	Completion of tuberculosis therapy
Functional status preservation and rehabilitation	Improvement in ambulation in home health care patients
Functional status preservation and rehabilitation	Nursing home residents needing more help with daily activities
Supportive and palliative care	Shortness of breath among home health care patients
Supportive and palliative care	Pressure sores in nursing home residents

* Noncore measure.

Management

Some diseases, such as diabetes and end stage renal disease, are chronic, which means they cannot simply be treated once; they must be managed across a lifetime. Management of chronic disease often involves promotion and maintenance of lifestyle changes and regular contact with a provider to monitor the status of the disease. For patients, effective management of chronic diseases can mean the difference between normal, healthy living and frequent medical problems.

Outcomes

Many factors other than health care influence health outcomes, including a person's genes, lifestyle, and social and physical environment. However, for many individuals, appropriate preventive services, timely treatment of acute illness and injury, and meticulous management of chronic disease can positively affect mortality, morbidity, and quality of life.

The measures highlighted in this chapter are categorized as follows:

Cancer

Importance

Mortality

Number of deaths (2009).. 562,340[1]

Cause of death rank (2006) ....2nd[2]

Prevalence

Number of living Americans who have been diagnosed with cancer (2005)...... ....11,098,450[3]

Incidence

New cases of cancer (2009) ....1,479,350[1]

New cases of breast cancer in women (2009)............................192,370[1]

Cost

Total cost[IX] (2008 est.) ....$243.4 billion[4]

Indirect costs (2008 est.).. $144.4 billion[4]

Direct costs (2008 est.) .... $99 billion[4]

Cost-effectiveness[X] of breast cancer screening .... $35,000-$165,000/QALY[5]

Measures

Evidence-based consensus defining good quality care and how to measure it currently exists for only a few cancers and a few aspects of care. Breast and colorectal cancers have high incidence rates and are highlighted in alternate years of the report. The 2008 *National Healthcare Quality Report* (NHQR) highlighted colorectal cancer; this year's focus is on breast cancer. The core report measures are:

- Breast cancer screening (mammography).
- Breast cancer first diagnosed at advanced stage.
- Breast cancer deaths.

As in previous reports, the 2009 NHQR includes two noncore measures for breast cancer care from the National Cancer Data Base that have been endorsed by the National Quality Forum:

- Women with clinical Stage I-IIb breast cancer who received either axillary node dissection or sentinel lymph node biopsy at the time of surgery.
- Women under age 70 treated with breast-conserving surgery who received radiation therapy within 1 year of diagnosis.

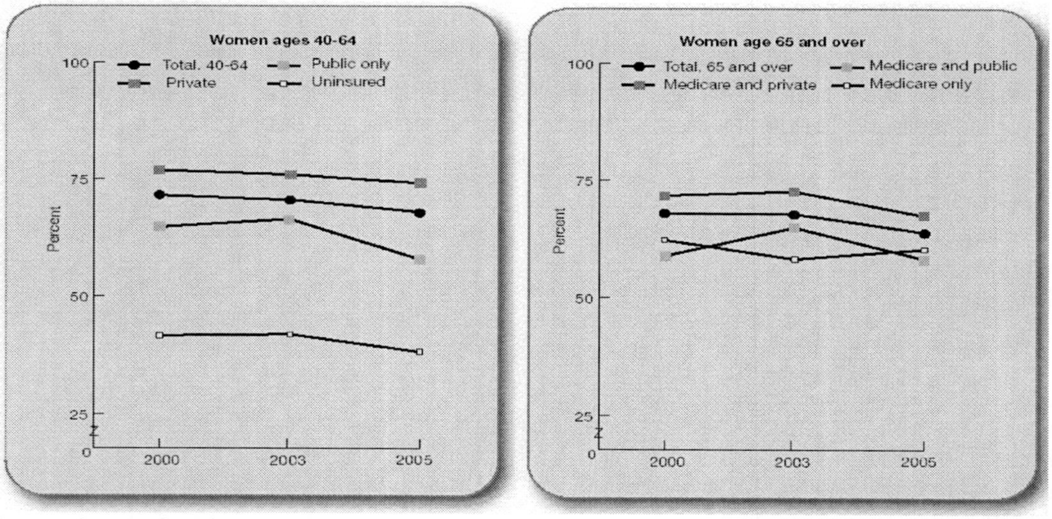

Source: Centers for Disease Control and Prevention, National Center for Health Statistics, National Health Interview Survey, 2000, 2003, and 2005.

Denominator: Civilian noninstitutionalized women age 40 and over.

Note: Insurance-specific rates are age adjusted to the 2000 U.S. standard population.

Figure 2.1. Women age 40 and over who reported they had a mammogram within the past 2 years, by insurance status, 2000, 2003, and 2005

Findings

Prevention: Breast Cancer Screening (Mammography)

Early detection of cancer increases treatment options and often improves outcomes. Mammography, the most effective method for detecting breast cancer at its early stages,[6] can identify malignancies before they can be felt and before symptoms develop. For available data years, the U.S. Preventive Services Task Force recommended mammograms every 1 to 2 years for women age 40 and over.[7]

- The percentage of women ages 40-64 who reported they had a mammogram in the past 2 years decreased from 71.5% in 2000 to 67.9% in 2005 (Figure 2.1).
- The percentage of women ages 40-64 with public insurance only who had a mammogram decreased from 64.7% in 2000 to 57.9% in 2005, while rates did not change significantly for privately insured or uninsured women.
- In all 3 years, uninsured women and women with public insurance only ages 40-64 were less likely to have a mammogram than privately insured women.
- The percentage of women age 65 and over who reported they had a mammogram in the past 2 years decreased from 67.9% in 2000 to 63.8% in 2005.
- In all 3 years, women with Medicare and public insurance and women with Medicare only were less likely to have a mammogram than women with Medicare and private supplemental insurance.[XI]

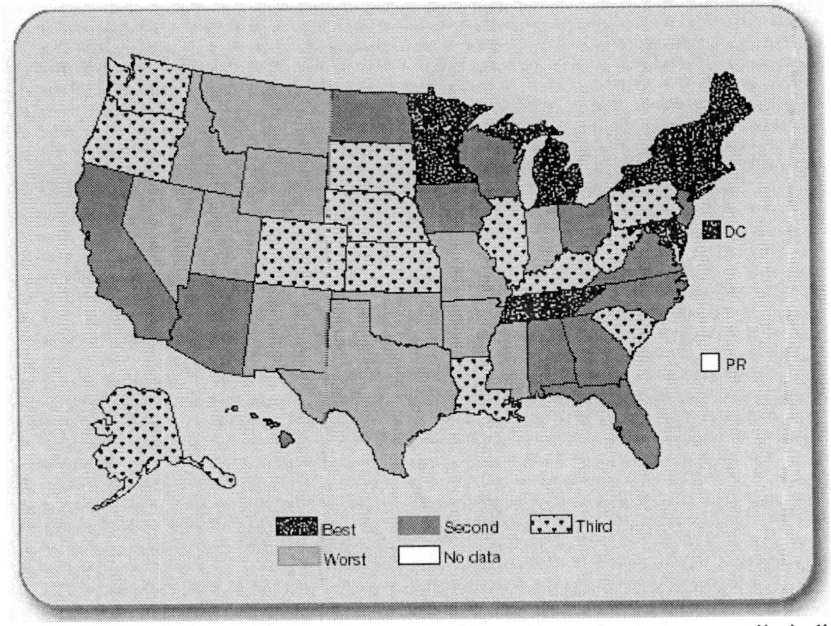

Key: Best quartile indicates States with highest rates of mammography; worst quartile indicates States with lowest rates.

Source: Centers for Disease Control and Prevention, Behavioral Risk Factor Surveillance System, 2006.

Figure 2.2. State variation: Women age 40 and over who reported they had a mammogram within the past 2 years, 2006

- The percentage of women age 65 and over with Medicare and private supplemental insurance who had a mammogram decreased from 71.7% in 2000 to 67.4% in 2005, while rates did not change significantly for women with Medicare and public insurance or Medicare only.
- Twelve States[XII] and the District of Columbia were in the best quartile (highest rates of mammography) in 2006 and had rates that ranged from 79.0% to 84.8%. All New England States are included in this quartile (Figure 2.2).
- The 12 States[XIII] in the worst quartile (lowest rates) in 2006 had rates of mammography that ranged from 66.7% to 71.4%. These States are primarily located in the West South Central and Mountain areas.

Outcome: Advanced Stage Breast Cancer

Cancers can be diagnosed at different stages of development. Cancers diagnosed early before spread has occurred are generally more amenable to treatment and cure; cancers diagnosed late with extensive spread often have poor prognoses. The rate of cancer cases that are diagnosed at late or advanced stages is a measure of the effectiveness of cancer screening efforts and of adherence to followup care after a positive screening test. Because many cancers often take years to develop, changes in rates of late-stage cancer may lag behind changes in rates of screening.

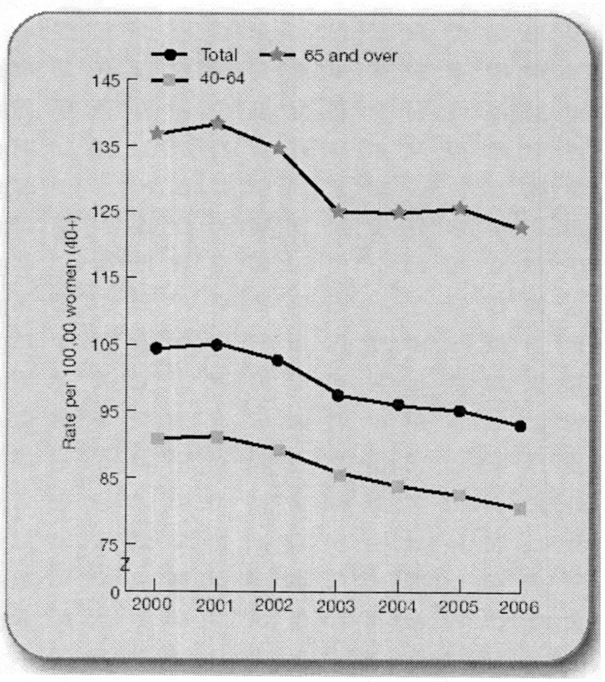

Source: National Cancer Institute, Surveillance, Epidemiology, and End Results Program, 2000-2006.
Denominator: Women age 40 and over.
Note: Age adjusted to the 2000 U.S. standard population. Advanced stage breast cancer is defined as local stage with tumor size greater than 2 cm diameter, regional stage, or distant stage.

Figure 2.3. Age-adjusted rate of advanced stage breast cancer per 100,000 women age 40 and over, by age, 2000-2006

- Between 2000 and 2006, the overall rate of advanced stage breast cancer in women age 40 and over decreased from 104.3 to 92.9 per 100,000 women (Figure 2.3).
- From 2000 to 2006, the rate of advanced stage breast cancer in women ages 40-64 decreased from 90.8 to 80.6 per 100,000 women. During the same period, women age 65 and over also saw a decrease, from 136.8 to 122.5 per 100,000 women. These decreases may reflect improvements in mammography rates during the 1990s.
- In all years, women age 65 and over had higher rates of advanced stage breast cancer than women ages 40-64.

Treatment: Receipt of Recommended Care for Breast Cancer

Different diagnostic and treatment options exist for various types of cancer. Some aspects of cancer care are well established as beneficial and are commonly recommended. The appropriateness of recommended care depends on different factors, such as the stage or the extent of the cancer within the body (especially whether the disease has spread from the original site to other parts of the body). Other types of care are important for accurate diagnosis, such as ensuring adequate examination of lymph nodes when surgery is performed.

- The percentage of women under age 65 with clinical Stage I-IIb breast cancer who received axillary node dissection or sentinel lymph node biopsy at the time of surgery (lumpectomy or mastectomy) increased from 78.0% in 2000 to 87.8% in 2006 (Figure 2.4). Improvement was observed among all insurance groups.

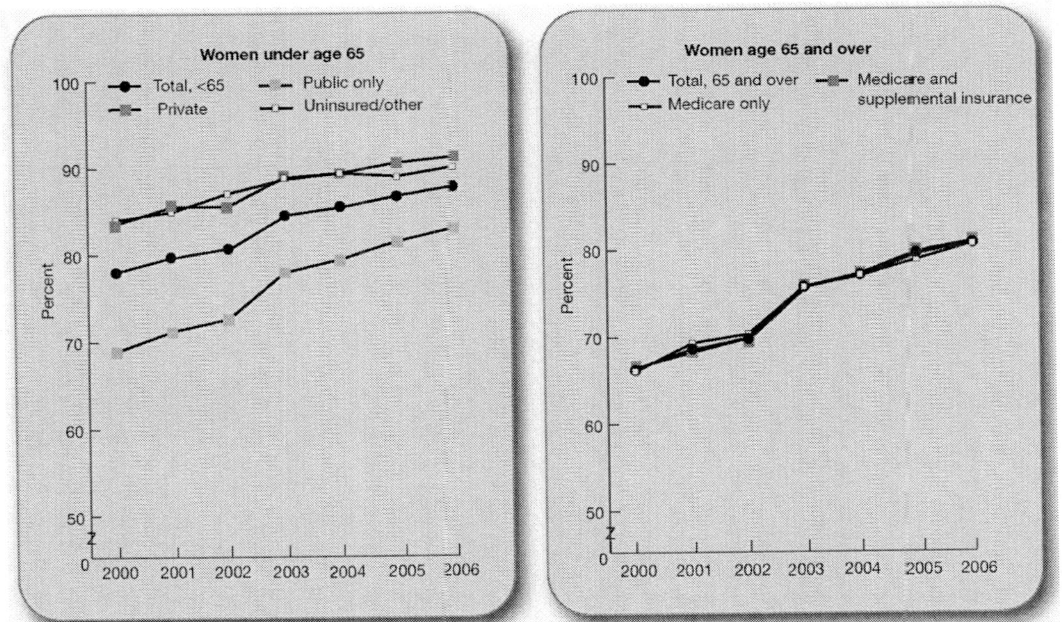

Source: Commission on Cancer, American College of Surgeons and American Cancer Society, National Cancer Data Base, 2000-2006.

Denominator: U.S. population, women with Stage I-IIb breast cancer.

Figure 2.4. Women with clinical Stage I-IIb breast cancer who received axillary node dissection or sentinel lymph node biopsy at the time of surgery (lumpectomy or mastectomy), by insurance status, 2000-2006

- In all years, women under age 65 with public health insurance only were less likely than those with private insurance to receive axillary node dissection or sentinel lymph node biopsy.
- Between 2000 and 2006, the percentage of women age 65 and over who received axillary node dissection or sentinel lymph node biopsy increased from 66.4% to 80.8%. Improvement was observed among both women with Medicare and supplemental insurance and women with Medicare only.
- In all years, women age 65 and over with Medicare only and with Medicare and supplemental insurance had similar rates of axillary node dissection or sentinel lymph node biopsy.
- Between 2000 and 2006, the percentage of women under age 65 treated for breast cancer with breast-conserving surgery who received radiation therapy to the breast within 1 year of diagnosis remained stable with no statistically significant changes (Figure 2.5).
- In 2006, uninsured women under age 65 were less likely than women with private insurance to receive radiation therapy following breast-conserving surgery.
- Between 2000 and 2006, the percentage of women ages 65-69 treated for breast cancer with breast-conserving surgery who received radiation therapy to the breast within 1 year of diagnosis remained stable with no statistically significant changes.
- In all years, women ages 65-69 with Medicare only were less likely than those with Medicare and supplemental insurance to receive radiation therapy.

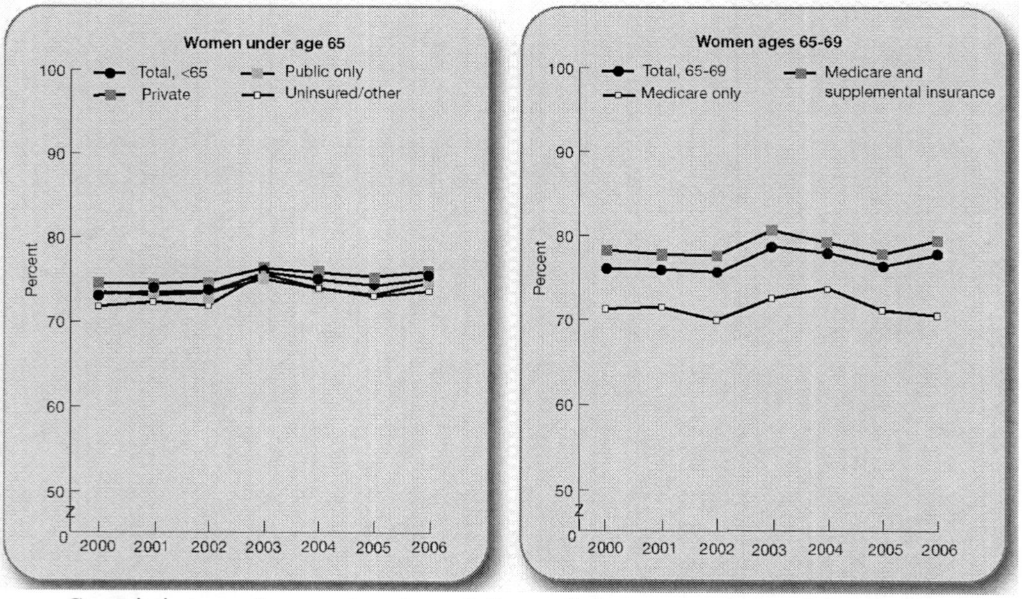

Source: Commission on Cancer, American College of Surgeons and American Cancer Society, National Cancer Data Base, 2000-2006.

Denominator: U.S. population, women under age 70 treated for breast cancer (American Joint Committee on Cancer Stage I, II, or III primary invasive epithelial breast cancer) with breast-conserving surgery.

Figure 2.5. Women under age 70 treated for breast cancer with breast-conserving surgery who received radiation therapy to the breast within 1 year of diagnosis, by insurance status, 2000-2006

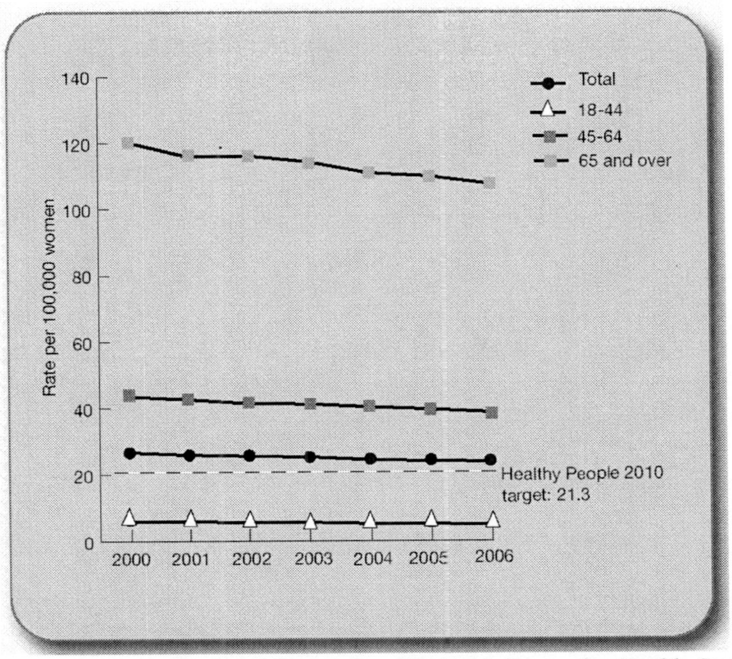

Source: Centers for Disease Control and Prevention, National Center for Health Statistics, National Vital Statistics System—Mortality, 2000-2006.
Denominator: U.S. population, women.
Note: Total rate is age adjusted to the 2000 U.S. standard population.

Figure 2.6. Age-adjusted breast cancer deaths per 100,000 women, by age, 2000-2006

Outcome: Breast Cancer Deaths

The death rate from a disease is a function of many factors, including the causes of the disease; social forces; and the effectiveness of the health care system in providing prevention, treatment, and management of the disease. Breastcancer deaths reflect the impact of breast cancer screening, diagnosis, and treatment. Mortality is measured as the number of deaths per 100,000 women. Declines in breast cancer deaths can be attributed, in part, to improvements in early detection and treatment.

- Between 2000 and 2006, the rate of breast cancer deaths decreased from 26.8 to 23.5 per 100,000 women (Figure 2.6).
- At 23.5 deaths per 100,000 women, the overall breast cancer death rate in 2006 was higher than the Healthy People 2010 target of 21.3. At the present rate of change, this target could be met by 2010.
- From 2000 to 2006, the rate of breast cancer deaths decreased significantly for all age groups.
- For all data years, women age 65 and over were more likely to die from breast cancer than those under age 65.

Diabetes

Importance

Mortality

Number of deaths (2006) ....72,449[2]
Cause of death rank (2006)...6th[2]

Prevalence

Total number of Americans with diabetes (2007)........................ 23.6 million[8]
Number of Americans diagnosed with diabetes (2007).................... 17.9 million[8]
Number of Americans with undiagnosed diabetes (2007)................. 5.7 million[8]

Incidence

New cases (age 20 and over, 2007)... 1.6 million[8]

Cost

Total cost (2007 est.).. $174 billion[9]
Direct medical costs (2007 est.) .... $116 billion[9]

Measures

Effective management of diabetes includes appropriate receipt of recommended processes, such as hemoglobin A1c (HbA1c)[XIV] tests, eye examinations, and foot examinations. Effective management also promotes outcomes expected to correlate positively with these processes, such as control of cholesterol, blood pressure, and HbA1c levels.

The core report measure highlighted in this section is:

- Receipt of three recommended diabetes services.

In addition, three noncore measures are presented:

- Control of HbA1c, cholesterol, and blood pressure.

Findings

Management: Receipt of Three Recommended Diabetes Services

The NHQR uses a composite measure to track the national rate of the receipt of all three recommended annual diabetes interventions: an HbA1c test, an eye examination, and a foot examination. These are basic process measures that provide an assessment of the quality of diabetes management.

- Between 2002 and 2006, the percentages of adults ages 40-64 and age 65 and over with diagnosed diabetes who received three recommended services for diabetes did not change significantly overall or for any insurance group (Figure 2.7).

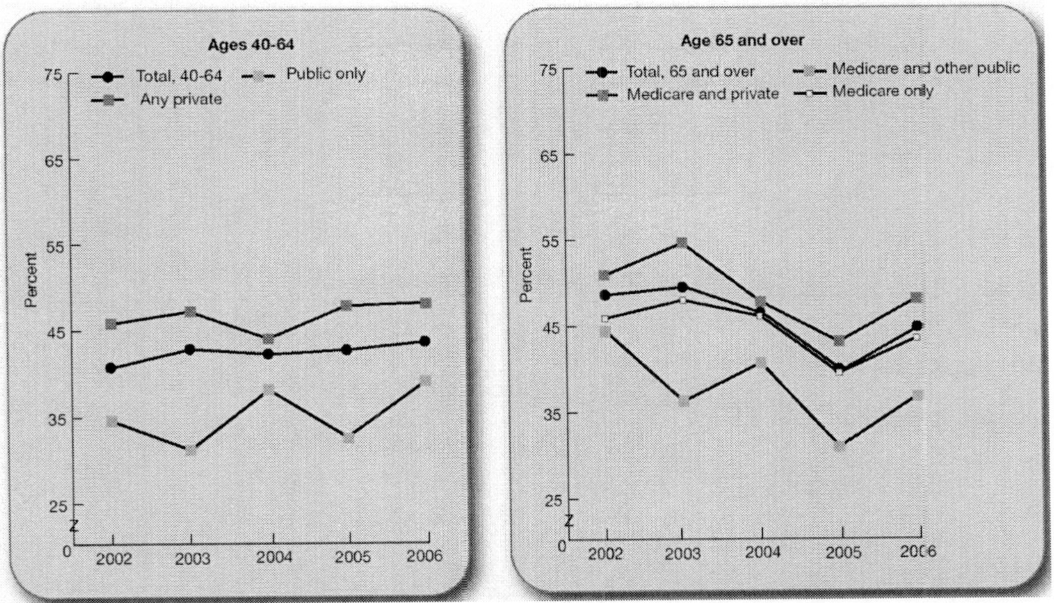

Source: Agency for Healthcare Research and Quality, Medical Expenditure Panel Survey, 2002-2006.
Denominator: Civilian noninstitutionalized population with diagnosed diabetes, age 40 and over.
Note: Data include people with both type 1 and type 2 diabetes.

Figure 2.7. Composite measure: Adults age 40 and over with diagnosed diabetes who received three recommended services for diabetes in the calendar year (hemoglobin A1c measurement, dilated eye examination, and foot examination), by insurance status, 2002-2006

- In 3 of 5 years, adults ages 40-64 with public insurance were significantly less likely than those with private insurance to receive recommended services. In 2 of 5 years, adults age 65 and over with Medicare and other public insurance were significantly less likely than those with Medicare and private insurance to receive recommended services. There were no statistically significant differences between insurance groups in 2006.

Management and Outcome: Receipt of HbA1c Measurement and Admissions for Short-Term Diabetes Complications

This year, the NHQR introduces a new type of State variation map. Rather than focus on a single process or outcome measure, these maps seek to identify States that perform poorly on both a process measure and a related outcome measure. These maps do not imply causality; improvements in processes of care typically affect outcomes many years in the future. Rather, these maps are intended to help identify those States that may have the greatest opportunity to improve performance in this area.

For diabetes, HbA1c measurement is critical for guiding treatment and achieving good control of glucose. Individuals who do not achieve good control are more prone to develop diabetic ketoacidosis and other short-term complications requiring hospitalization.

- The 11 States[XV] in the worst quartile (lowest rate) in 2006 for patients with diagnosed diabetes who received an HbA1c measurement had rates that ranged from 70.6% to 79.9% (Figure 2.8).

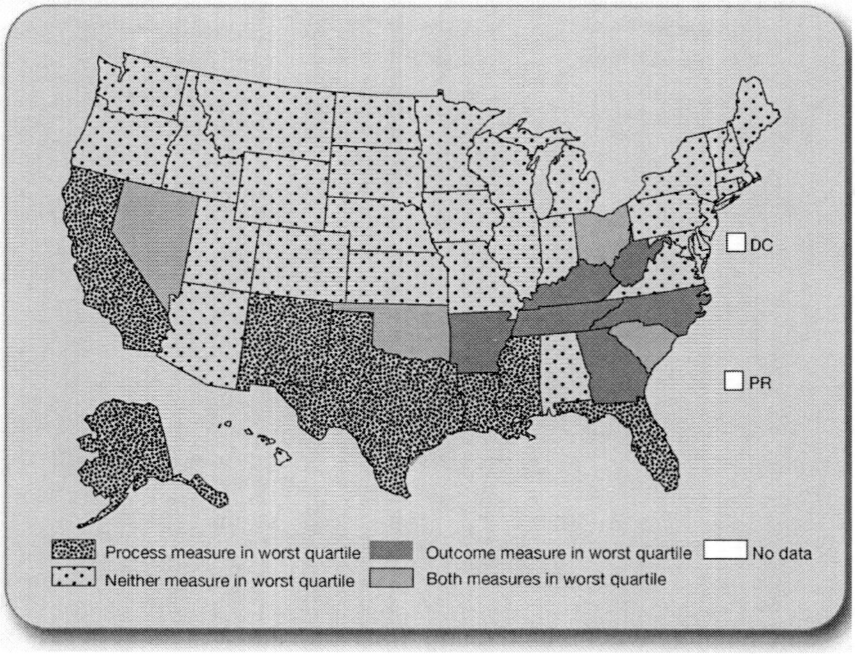

Key: Process measure in worst quartile indicates States with the lowest rates of HbA1c measurement; outcome measure in worst quartile indicates States with the highest rates of admission for short-term complications of diabetes.

Source: Centers for Disease Control and Prevention, Behavioral Risk Factor Surveillance System, 2006 (HbA1c measurement); Agency for Healthcare Research and Quality, Healthcare Cost and Utilization Project, 2006 (admissions for diabetes with short-term complications).

Figure 2.8. State variation: Adults age 40 and over with diagnosed diabetes who received a hemoglobin A1c measurement (2006) and admissions for diabetes with short-term complications per 100,000 population age 18 and over (2006)

- The 10 States[XVI] in the worst quartile (highest rate) in 2006 for admissions for diabetes with short-term complications had admission rates that ranged from 66.7 to 85.1 per 100,000 population age 18 and over.
- Four States[XVII] were in the worst quartile for both measures in 2006 with both low rates of HbA1c measurement among patients with diagnosed diabetes and high rates of admissions for diabetes with short-term complications.

Outcome: Controlled Hemoglobin, Cholesterol, and Blood Pressure

People diagnosed with diabetes are often at higher risk for other cardiovascular risk factors, such as high blood pressure and high cholesterol. Having these conditions in combination with diagnosed diabetes increases the likelihood of complications, such as heart and kidney diseases, blindness, nerve damage, and stroke. Patients who manage their diagnosed diabetes and maintain an HbA1c level of <7%, total cholesterol of <200 mg/dL, and blood pressure of <140/80 mm Hg[XVIII] can decrease these risks.

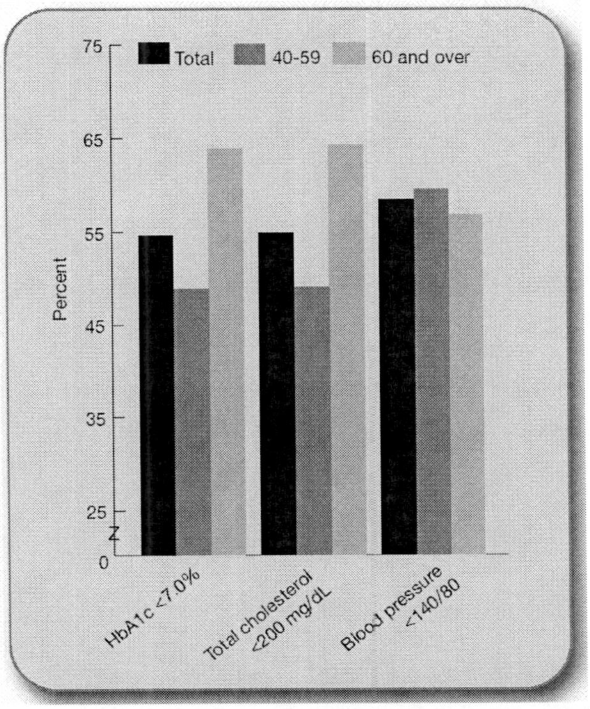

Source: Centers for Disease Control and Prevention, National Center for Health Statistics, National Health and Nutrition Examination Survey, 2003-2006.

Denominator: Civilian noninstitutionalized population with diagnosed diabetes, age 40 and over.

Note: Age adjusted to the 2000 U.S. standard population. Survey respondents were classified as having diabetes only if they had a previous diagnosis of diabetes from a doctor other than during a period of pregnancy (i.e., gestational diabetes was excluded). This is determined by a "Yes" response to the question: "Other than during pregnancy, have you ever been told by a doctor or health professional that you have diabetes or sugar diabetes?"

Figure 2.9. Adults age 40 and over with diagnosed diabetes with hemoglobin A1c, total cholesterol, and blood pressure under control, by age, 2003-2006

- In 2003-2006, only 54.6% of adults age 40 and over diagnosed with diabetes had their HbA1c level under optimal control (<7%) (Figure 2.9). Only 54.9% had total cholesterol <200, and only 58.5% had blood pressure <140/80.
- In 2003-2006, adults age 60 and over were more likely to have their HbA1c levels under optimal control compared with adults ages 40-59.
- In 2003-2006, adults age 60 and over were more likely to have cholesterol levels <200 mg/dL compared with adults ages 40-59.

End Stage Renal Disease

Importance

Mortality

Total end stage renal disease (ESRD) deaths (2006)...................................... 87,654[10]

Prevalence
Total cases (2006)......................... 506,256[10]

Incidence
Number of new cases (2006)....................................110,854[10]

Cost
Total ESRD Medicare program expenditures (2006 est.).....................$23.9 billion[11]

Measures

The NHQR includes six measures of ESRD management to assess the quality of care provided to renal dialysis patients. The two core report measures highlighted here are:

- Adequacy of hemodialysis.
- Registration for transplantation.

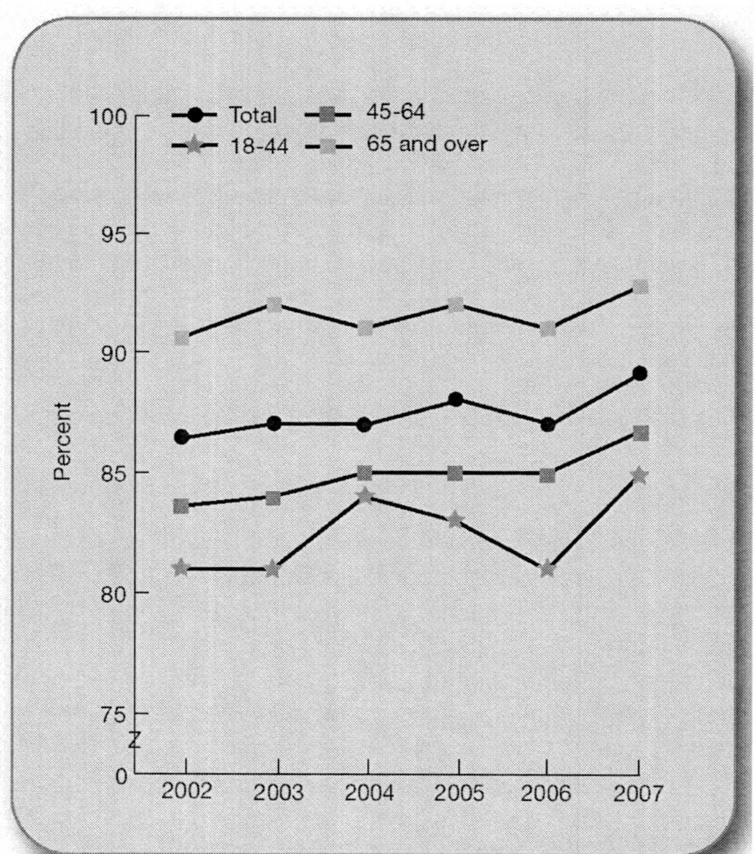

Source: Centers for Medicare & Medicaid Services, ESRD Clinical Performance Measures Project, 2002-2007.
Denominator: ESRD hemodialysis patients age 18 and over.

Figure 2.10. Adult hemodialysis patients with adequate dialysis (urea reduction ratio 65% or greater), by age, 2002-2007

Findings

Outcome: Adequate Hemodialysis

Dialysis removes harmful waste and excess fluid buildup in the blood that occurs when kidneys fail to function. Hemodialysis is the most common method used to treat advanced and permanent kidney failure. The adequacy of dialysis is measured by the percentage of hemodialysis patients with a urea reduction ratio equal to or greater than 65%; this measure indicates how well urea, a waste product, is eliminated by the dialysis machine.

- From 2002 to 2007, the percentage of adult hemodialysis patients receiving adequate dialysis improved from 86.4% to 89.2% (Figure 2.10). Improvements were observed among all age groups.
- In all years, adults ages 18-44 and 45-64 were less likely than adults age 65 and over to receive adequate dialysis.

Management: Registration for Transplantation

Kidney transplantation is a procedure that replaces a failing kidney with a healthy kidney. If a patient is deemed a good candidate for transplant, he or she is placed on the transplant program's waiting list. Dialysis patients wait for transplant centers to match them with the most suitable donor. Registration for transplantation is an initial step toward patients receiving the option of kidney transplantation. Patients who receive transplants from living donors, about 36% of kidney transplants, do not need to register on a waiting list.

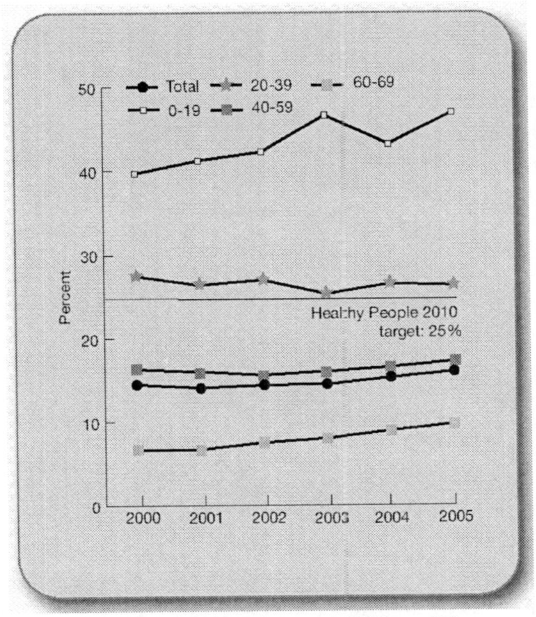

Source: National Institute of Diabetes and Digestive and Kidney Diseases, U.S. Renal Data System, 2000-2005.

Denominator: ESRD hemodialysis patients and peritoneal dialysis patients under age 70.

Figure 2.11. Dialysis patients who were registered on a waiting list for transplantation, by age, 2000-2005

Early transplantation that decreases or eliminates the need for dialysis can also lessen the occurrence of acute rejection and patient mortality. In 2006, 70,778 patients were on the Organ Procurement and Transplantation Network's deceased donor kidney transplant waiting list in the United States. Only 10,212 deceased donor kidney transplants were performed.[12]

- From 2000 to 2005, the percentage of dialysis patients who were registered on a waiting list for transplantation improved from 14.5% to 16.0% (Figure 2.11). Improvements were observed among all age groups except patients ages 20-39.
- In all years, patients ages 20-69 were less likely to be registered on a waiting list compared with patients ages 0-19.
- Registration rates among patients ages 0-39 exceeded the Healthy People 2010 target of 25.0%, while rates among other age groups were not on track to meet this target.
- The 13 States[XIX] in the best quartile (highest rates of registration on a waiting list) in 2005 (Figure 2.12) had rates of registration that ranged from 19.9% to 28.7%. These States are primarily located in the Northeast and Midwest.
- Eleven States,[XX] the District of Columbia, and Puerto Rico were in the worst quartile (lowest rates) in 2005 and had rates of registration that ranged from 5.9% to 11.1%. These States are primarily located in the South.

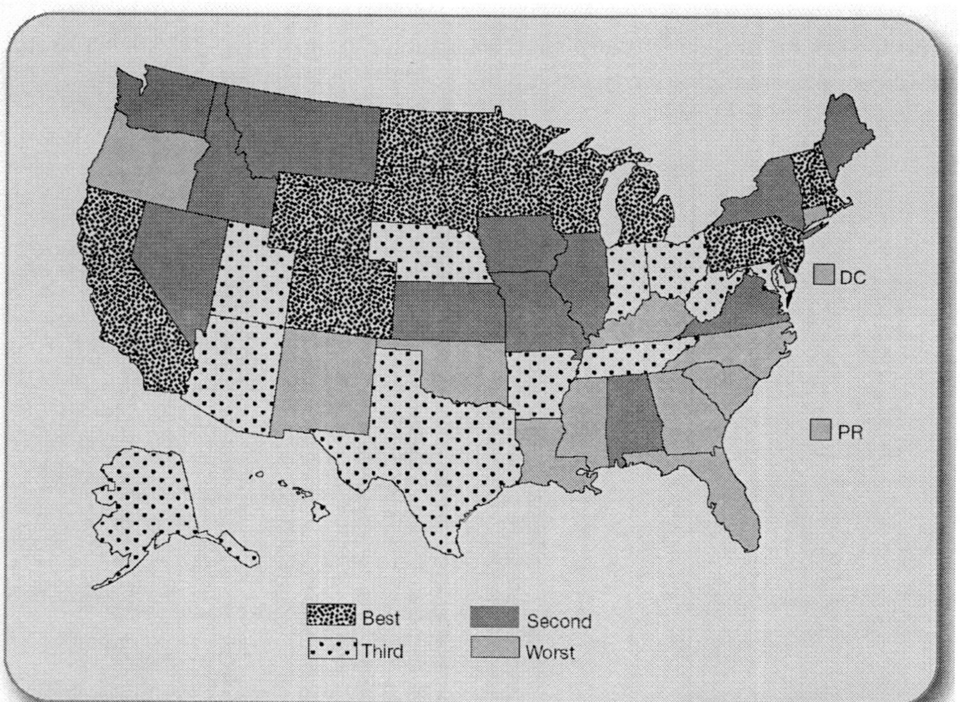

Key: Best quartile indicates States with highest rates of registration on a waiting list; worst quartile indicates States with lowest rates.

Source: National Institute of Diabetes and Digestive and Kidney Diseases, U.S. Renal Data System, 2005.

Figure 2.12. State variation: Dialysis patients who were registered on a waiting list for transplantation, 2005

Heart Disease

Importance

Mortality

Number of deaths (2006)..631,636[2]

Cause of death rank (2006)....................................1st[2]

Prevalence

Number of cases of coronary heart disease (2006)............ 16.8 million[13]

Number of cases of heart failure (2006)............................ 5.7 million[13]

Number of cases of high blood pressure (2006).......................... 73.6 million[13]

Number of heart attacks (2006).................................... 7.9 million[13]

Incidence

Number of new cases of heart failure (2004)........................ 550,000[14]

Cost

Total cost of cardiovascular disease (2009 est.)...................................... $474.8 billion[4]

Total cost of heart failure (2009 est.) ....$37.2 billion[13]

Direct costs of cardiovascular disease (2009 est.) .... $313.3 billion[4]

Cost-effectiveness of hypertension screening............. $14,000-$35,000/QALY[5]

Measures

The NHQR tracks several quality measures for preventing and treating heart disease, including the following three core report measures:

- Receipt of angiotensin-converting enzyme (ACE) inhibitor or angiotensin receptor blocker (ARB) for heart attack.
- Inpatient deaths following heart attack.
- Receipt of recommended care for heart failure.

Several measures related to heart disease are also presented in other sections of this chapter. Timeliness of cardiac reperfusion for heart attack patients is tracked in Chapter 4, Timeliness, and receipt of complete written discharge instructions by patients with heart failure is tracked in Chapter 5, Patient Centeredness.

Findings

Treatment: Receipt of Angiotensin-Converting Enzyme Inhibitor or Angiotensin Receptor Blocker for Heart Attack

Heart attack or acute myocardial infarction is a common life-threatening condition that requires rapid recognition and efficient treatment in a hospital to reduce the risk of serious heart damage and death. Measuring processes of heart attack care can provide information about whether a patient received specific needed services, but these processes make up a very small proportion of all the care that a heart attack patient needs. Measuring outcomes of heart attack care, such as mortality, can provide a more global assessment of all the care a patient receives and usually is the aspect of quality that matters most to patients.

Significant improvements in a number of measures of quality of care for heart attack have occurred in recent years. Four measures that have been tracked in past NHQRs (administration of aspirin within 24 hours and at discharge, administration of beta blocker at discharge, and counseling to quit smoking) have attained overall performance levels exceeding 95%. These measures were included in the composite measure of care for heart attack in past NHQRs. However, the success of these measures creates a ceiling effect that limits the report's ability to track improvement over time. In addition, administration of beta blocker within 24 hours has been discontinued. Hence, this NHQR focuses on one measure of heart attack care, ACE inhibitor or ARB treatment among patients with left ventricular systolic dysfunction.

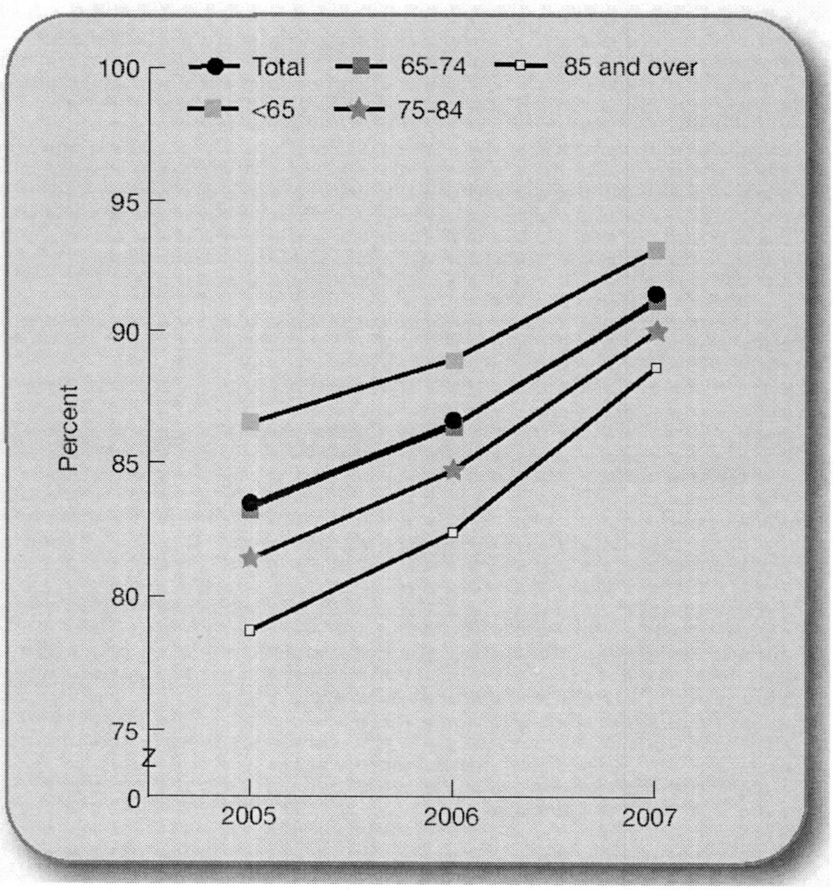

Key: ACE = angiotensin-converting enzyme; ARB = angiotensin receptor blocker.

Source: Centers for Medicare & Medicaid Services, Medicare Quality Improvement Organization Program, 2005-2007.

Denominator: Patients hospitalized with a principal diagnosis of acute myocardial infarction and left ventricular systolic dysfunction.

Figure 2.13. Hospital patients with heart attack and left ventricular systolic dysfunction who received ACE inhibitor or ARB, by age, 2005-2007

- From 2005 to 2007, the percentage of heart attack patients with left ventricular systolic dysfunction who received an ACE inhibitor or ARB improved from 83.4% to 91.3% (Figure 2.13). Improvements over time were observed among all age groups.
- In all years, patients ages 65-74, 75-84, and 85 and over were less likely than patients under age 65 to receive ACE inhibitor or ARB treatment.

Outcome: Inpatient Deaths Following Heart Attack

Survival following admission for heart attack reflects multiple patient factors, such as a patient's comorbidities, as well as health care system factors, such as the possible need to transfer patients to other hospitals in order to receive services. It also may partly reflect receipt of appropriate health services.

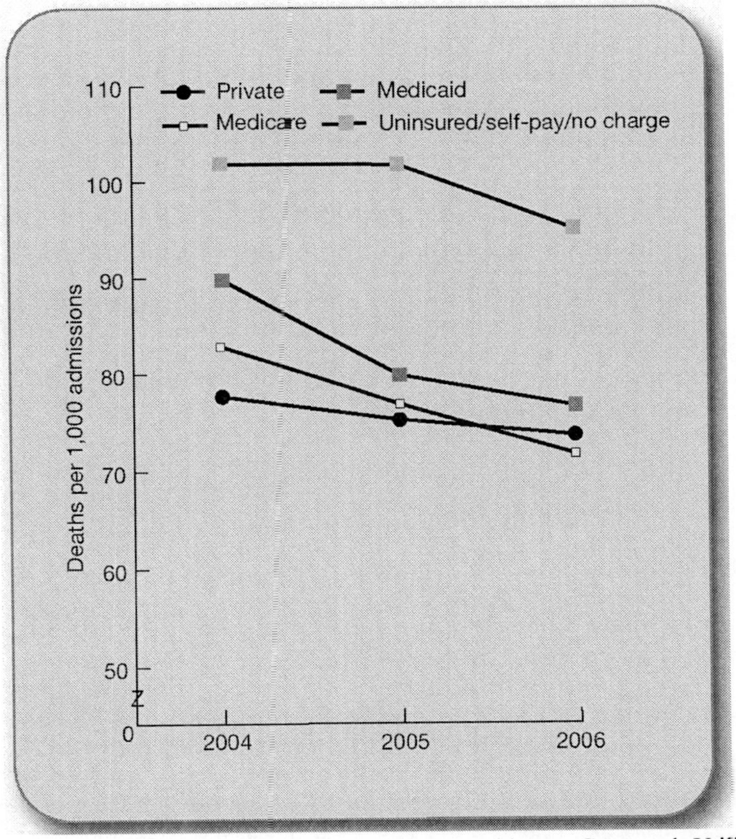

Source: Agency for Healthcare Research and Quality, Healthcare Cost and Utilization Project, Nationwide Inpatient Sample, 2004-2006.

Denominator: Adults age 18 and over admitted to a non-Federal community hospital in the United States with acute myocardial infarction as principal discharge diagnosis.

Note: Rates are adjusted by age, gender, age-gender interactions, and all payer refined-diagnosis related group scoring of risk of mortality.

Figure 2.14. Deaths per 1,000 adult hospital admissions with heart attack, by insurance status, 2004-2006

- Between 2004 and 2006, the overall inpatient mortality rate decreased significantly for those with private insurance, Medicare, Medicaid, and no insurance (Figure 2.14).
- In all 3 years, death rates among uninsured/self-pay/no charge patients were higher than among patients with private insurance.

Treatment and Outcome: Receipt of Angiotensin-Converting Enzyme Inhibitor or Angiotensin Receptor Blocker and Deaths per 1,000 Admissions With Heart Attack

Figure 2.15 shows States that perform poorly on both a process measure and an outcome measure related to heart attack. As noted earlier, these maps are intended to help identify those States that may have the greatest opportunity to improve performance in this area. For heart attacks, receipt of ACE inhibitor or ARB when indicated may be a marker of better cardiac care overall. Greater compliance with recommended care for heart attack may be associated with better outcomes.

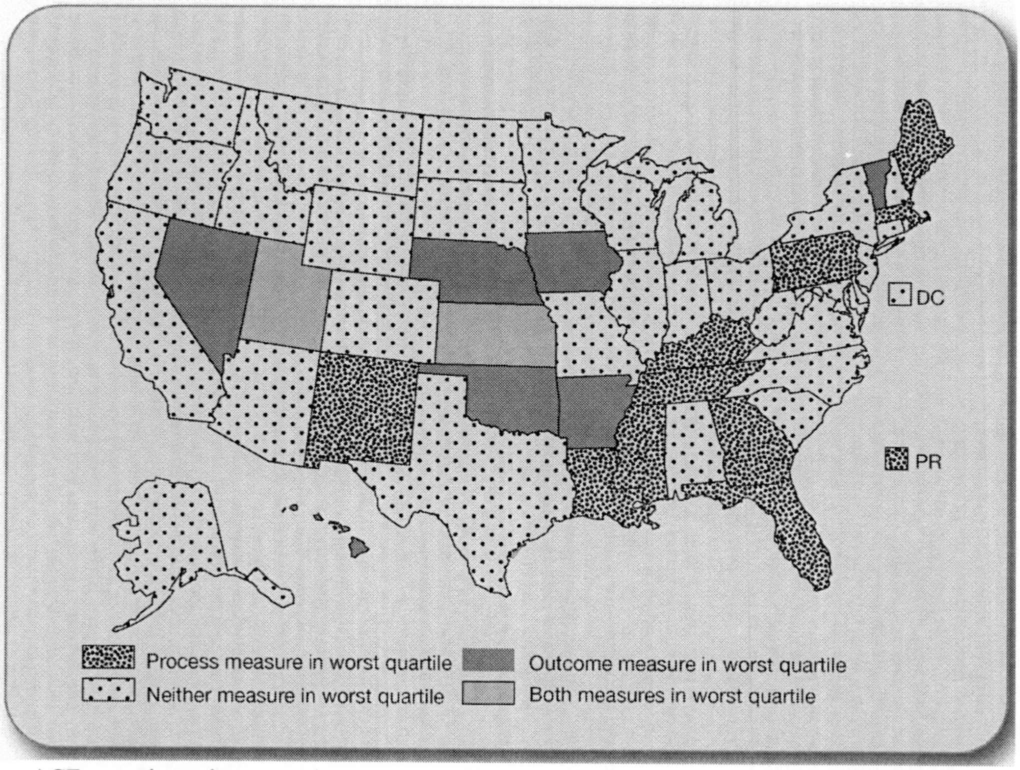

Key: ACE = angiotensin-converting enzyme; ARB = angiotensin receptor blocker. Process measure in worst quartile indicates States with the lowest rates of ACE inhibitor or ARB treatment; outcome measure in worst quartile indicates States with the highest inpatient death rates for acute myocardial infarction.

Source: Centers for Medicare & Medicaid Services, Medicare Quality Improvement Organization Program, 2007 (ACE inhibitor or ARB); Agency for Healthcare Research and Quality, Healthcare Cost and Utilization Project, 2006 (heart attack deaths).

Figure 2.15. State variation: Heart attack patients with left ventricular systolic dysfunction who received ACE inhibitor or ARB (2007) and deaths per 1,000 admissions wit h heart attack (2006)

- Twelve States[XXI] and Puerto Rico were in the worst quartile (lowest rates) for heart attack patients with left ventricular systolic dysfunction who received ACE inhibitor or ARB in 2007 (Figure 2.15). Among these areas, receipt of an ACE inhibitor or ARB ranged from 80.1% to 90.2%.
- Nine States[XXII] were in the worst quartile (highest rates) for deaths per 1,000 admissions with heart attack in 2006. Among these States, inpatient mortality ranged from 82.9 to 96.2 deaths per 1,000 admissions.
- Two States[XXIII] were in the worst quartile for both measures with both low rates of receipt of ACE inhibitor or ARB and high rates of deaths per 1,000 admissions for heart attack.

Treatment: Receipt of Recommended Care for Heart Failure

The NHQR tracks the national rates of receipt of the following services:

- Recommended test for heart functioning (heart failure patients having evaluation of left ventricular ejection fraction).
- Recommended medication treatment (patients with left ventricular systolic dysfunction prescribed ACE inhibitor or ARB at discharge).

In addition, an overall composite measure describes the percentage of all episodes in which heart failure patients receive recommended care.

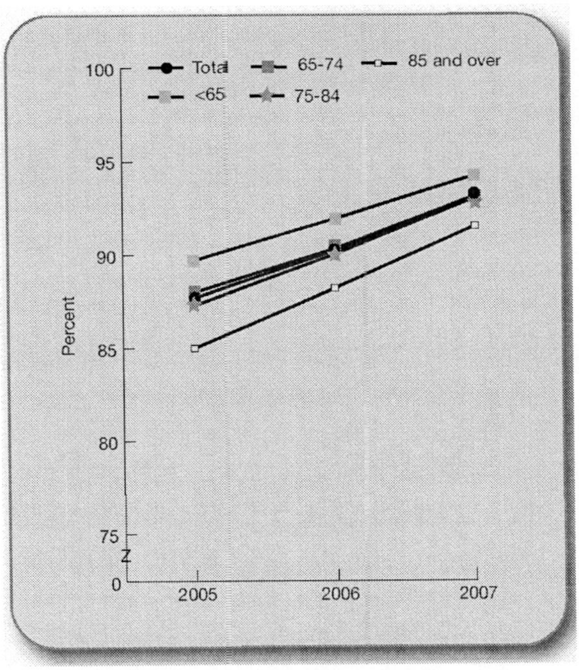

Source: Centers for Medicare & Medicaid Services, Medicare Quality Improvement Organization Program, 2005-2007.

Denominator: Patients hospitalized with a principal diagnosis of acute heart failure.

Figure 2.16. Hospital patients with heart failure who received recommended hospital care: Overall composite, by age, 2005-2007

- In 2007, 93.1% of recommended hospital care was received by patients hospitalized for heart failure (Figure 2.16).
- From 2005 to 2007, the percentage of recommended hospital care received improved overall and for all age groups.

HIV and AIDS

Importance

Mortality

Number of deaths of people with AIDS (2007).....................................14,561[15]

Prevalence

Number of people living with HIV infection (not including those with AIDS) (2007)........ 263,936[15]

Number of people living with AIDS (2007)..468,578[15]

Incidence

Number of new HIV infections (2007)........................56,300[15]

Number of new AIDS cases (2007)...............................37,041[15]

Cost

Federal spending on HIV/AIDS[XXIV](fiscal year 2009 est.) ....$19.4 billion[16]

Measures

This section highlights one core report measure focusing on quality of preventive care for HIV-infected individuals:

- New AIDS cases.

In addition, three noncore measures are presented on the prevention of opportunistic infections in AIDS patients and on HIV infection deaths:

- Eligible AIDS patients receiving prophylaxis for *Pneumocystis* pneumonia (PCP).
- Eligible AIDS patients receiving prophylaxis for *Mycobacterium avium* complex (MAC).
- HIV infection deaths.

Findings

Outcome: New AIDS Cases

Changes in HIV infection rates reflect changes in behavior by at-risk individuals that may only partly be influenced by the health care system. However, individual and community programs have shown progress in influencing behavior change. Changes in the incidence of new AIDS cases are affected by changes in HIV infection rates, screening and early detection of HIV disease, and availability of appropriate treatments for HIV-infected individuals. Improved treatments that extend life for those with the disease are reflected in the decrease in deaths due to AIDS from about 18,000 to 14,600 between 2003 and 2007, after showing no change for the previous 3 years.[17]

- The overall rate of new AIDS cases per 100,000 population decreased between 2000 and 2007 (16.8 to 14.4) (Figure 2.17).
- From 2000 to 2007, the rate of new AIDS cases also decreased for people ages 18-44 (24.5 to 19.9).
- The 2007 national rate of 14.4 new AIDS cases per 100,000 population is well above the Healthy People 2010 target of 1.0 new case per 100,000 population. If current trends continue, this target will not be met.

Management: PCP and MAC Prophylaxis

Management of chronic HIV disease includes outpatient and inpatient services. Without adequate treatment, as HIV disease progresses, CD4 cell counts fall and patients become increasingly susceptible to opportunistic infections. When CD4 cell counts fall below 200, medicine to prevent development of PCP is routinely recommended. When CD4 cell counts fall below 50, medicine to prevent development of disseminated MAC infection is routinely recommended.[18]

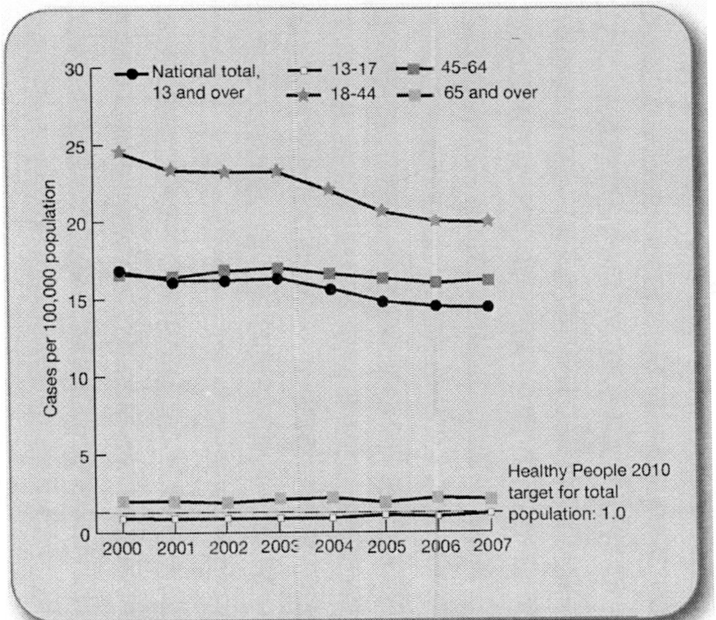

Source: Centers for Disease Control and Prevention, National Center for HIV, Viral Hepatitis, STD, and TB Prevention, HIV/AIDS Reporting System, 2000-2007.

Denominator: U.S. population age 13 and over.

Note: Rates are age adjusted to the 2000 U.S. standard population.

Figure 2.17. New AIDS cases per 100,000 population age 13 and over, by age, 2000-2007

Because national data on HIV care are not routinely collected, HIV measures tracked in the NHQR come from the HIV Research Network, which consists of 18 medical practices across the United States that treat large numbers of patients living with HIV. Data from the voluntary HIV Research Network are not nationally representative of the level of care received by all Americans living with HIV. Network data represent only patients who are actually receiving care (about 14,000 HIV patients per year) and do not represent patients who do not receive care. Furthermore, data shown below are not representative of the HIV Research Network as a whole because they represent only a subset of network sites that have the best data.

The Ryan White HIV/AIDS Program is the largest Federal program dedicated to providing HIV-related services to individuals who otherwise could not afford these services. These include individuals who are uninsured or have inadequate insurance and cannot cover the costs of care on their own. This safety net program may help mitigate the effects of uninsurance on receipt of HIV care.

- Of eligible patients (2,052 AIDS patients with at least two CD4 cell counts below 200), 93.2% received PCP prophylaxis in 2006 (Figure 2.18). From 2004 to 2006, receipt of PCP prophylaxis improved overall and for all insurance groups.

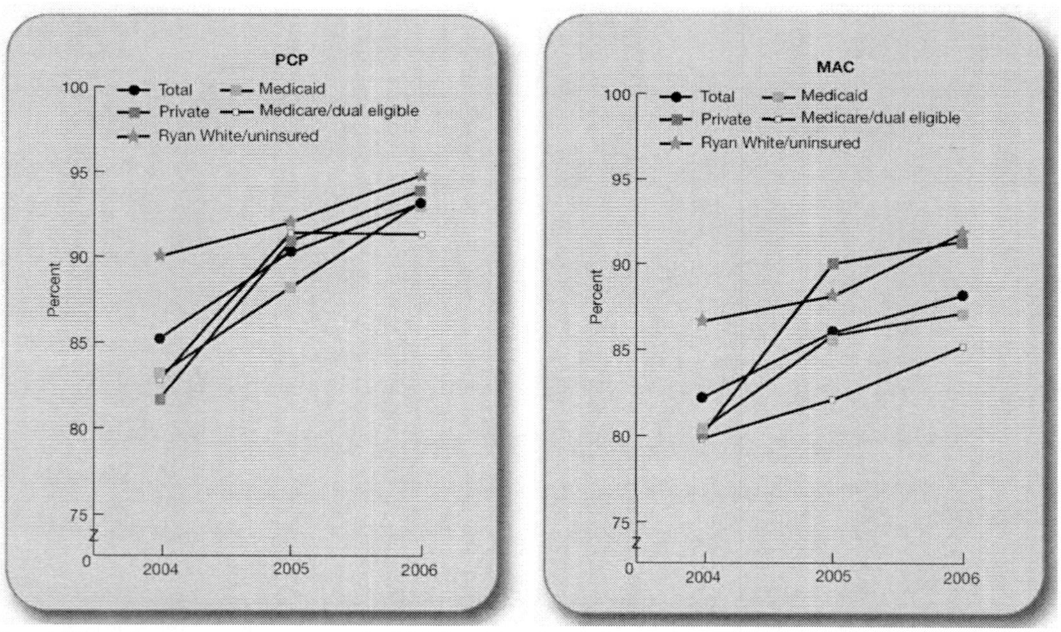

Key: PCP = *Pneumocystis* pneumonia; MAC = *Mycobacterium avium* complex.

Source: Agency for Healthcare Research and Quality, HIV Research Network, 2004-2006.

Denominator: Adult patients with HIV receiving care from an HIV Research Network medical practice who have CD4 cell counts below 200 (PCP) or below 50 (MAC).

Figure 2.18. Eligible adult AIDS patients receiving PCP and MAC prophylaxis in the calendar year, by insurance, 2004-2006

- In 2004, eligible patients with private insurance, Medicare, or Medicaid were less likely to receive PCP prophylaxis than those who were uninsured or receiving services funded by the Ryan White Program. In 2006, only patients with Medicare were significantly less likely to receive PCP prophylaxis than patients who were uninsured or received assistance through the Ryan White HIV/AIDS Program.
- Of eligible patients (594 AIDS patients with at least two CD4 cell counts below 50), 88.2% received MAC prophylaxis in 2006. From 2004 to 2006, receipt of MAC prophylaxis improved among patients with Medicaid.
- For all years, there were no statistically significant differences between insurance groups in receipt of MAC prophylaxis.

Outcome: HIV Infection Deaths

HIV infection deaths reflect a number of factors, including underlying rates of HIV risk behaviors, prevention of HIV transmission, early detection and treatment of HIV disease, and management of AIDS and its complications.

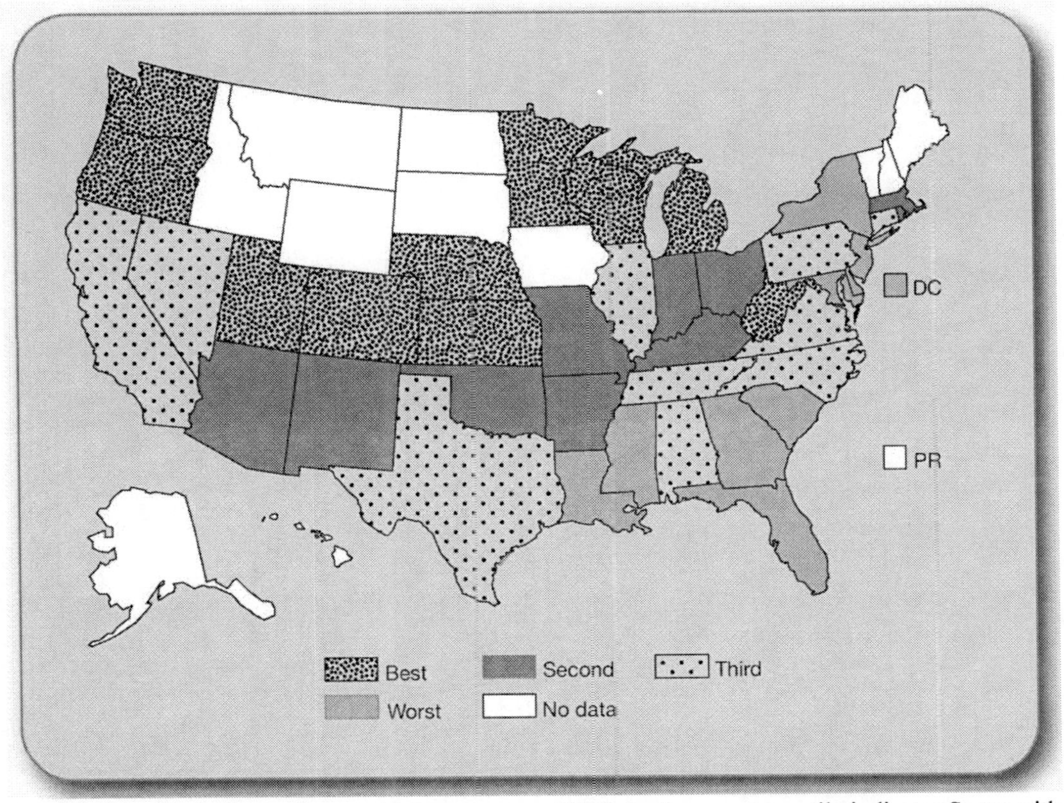

Key: Best quartile indicates States with lowest rates of HIV deaths; worst quartile indicates States with highest rates.

Source: Centers for Disease Control and Prevention, National Center for Health Statistics, National Vital Statistics System—Mortality, 2006.

Denominator: U.S. population.

Note: Rates are age adjusted to the 2000 U.S. standard population.

Figure 2.19. State variation: HIV infection deaths per 100,000 population, 2006

- The 10 States[XXV] in the best quartile (lowest rates of HIV deaths) in 2006 had a combined average rate of 1.3 deaths per 100,000 population (Figure 2.19).
- Nine States[XXVI] and the District of Columbia were in the worst quartile (highest rates) in 2006 and had a combined average rate of 10.2 deaths per 100,000 population. These States are primarily located in the mid-Atlantic and the South.

Maternal and Child Health

Importance

Mortality

Number of maternal deaths (2006) ....569[2]
Number of infant deaths (2006) ....28,527[2]

Demographics

Number of children[XXVII] (2007)... 73,590,243[19]
Number of babies born in United States (2006 est.)...................... 4,265,555[20]

Cost

Total cost of health care for children (2002 est.) ...... $79 billion[21]
Cost-effectiveness of vision screening for children .... $0-$14,000/QALY[5]
Cost-effectiveness of childhood immunization series[XXVIII].................... Cost saving[5]

Measures

Throughout the report, the NHQR tracks several prevention and treatment measures related to maternal and child health care. The core report measures highlighted in this section are:

- Receipt of all recommended immunizations by young children.
- Dental visits for children.
- Counseling children or parents about physical activity.
- Counseling children or parents about healthy eating.

In addition, two noncore measures are presented:

- Obstetric trauma.
- Weight monitoring of overweight children.

Findings

Outcome: Obstetric Trauma

Childbirth and reproductive care are the most common reasons for women of childbearing age to use health care services. With more than 11,000 births each day in the United States, [20] childbirth is the most common reason for hospital admission. Obstetric trauma involving a severe tear to the vagina or surrounding tissues during delivery is a common complication of childbirth.

- From 2004 to 2006, rates of obstetric trauma with 3rd or 4th degree laceration decreased among all age groups (Figure 2.20).
- In all years, females younger than age 35 had higher rates of obstetric trauma compared with women ages 35-54. This may in part reflect lower rates of vaginal delivery and higher rates of cesarean delivery among women ages 35-54.

Prevention: Receipt of All Recommended Immunizations by Young Children

Immunizations are important for reducing mortality and morbidity. They protect recipients from illness and disability and protect others in the community who cannot be vaccinated. In 2006, recommended vaccines for children that should have been completed by ages 19-35 months included four doses of diphtheria-tetanus-pertussis vaccine, three doses of polio vaccine, one dose of measles-mumps-rubella vaccine, three doses of *Haemophilus influenzae* type B vaccine, and three doses of hepatitis B vaccine.

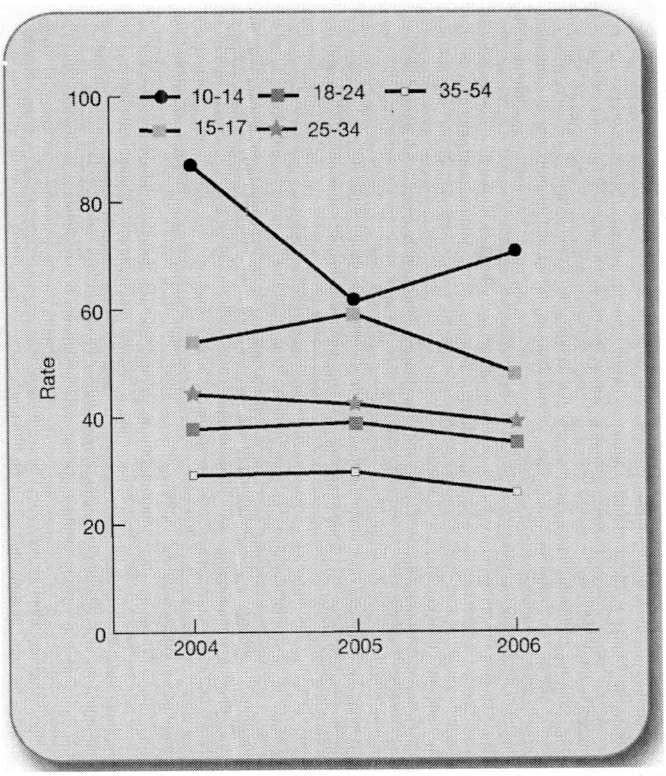

Source: Agency for Healthcare Research and Quality, Healthcare Cost and Utilization Project, Nationwide Inpatient Sample, 2004-2006.
Denominator: All patients hospitalized for vaginal delivery without indication of instrument assistance.
Note: Rates are not adjusted.

Figure 2.20. Obstetric trauma with 3rd or 4th degree laceration per 1,000 vaginal deliveries without instrument assistance, by age, 2004-2006

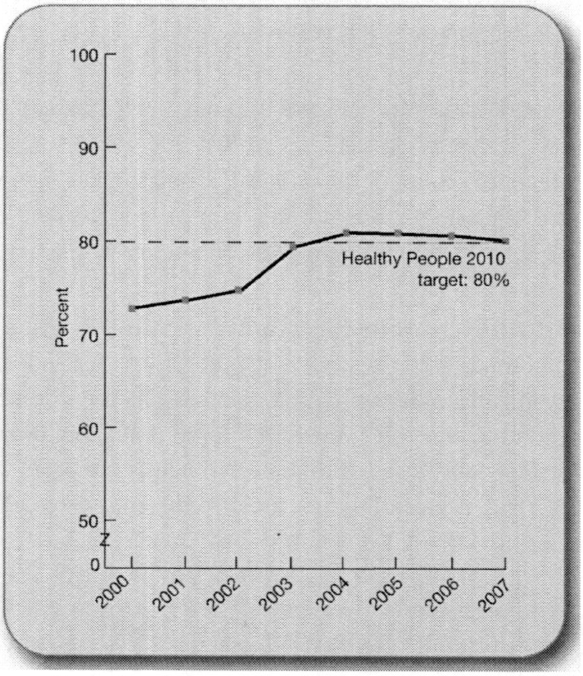

Source: Centers for Disease Control and Prevention, National Center for Health Statistics and National Center for Immunization and Respiratory Diseases, National Immunization Survey, 2000-2007.

Denominator: U.S. civilian noninstitutionalized population ages 19-35 months.

Note: The vaccines included in this measure are based on the corresponding Healthy People 2010 objective, which does not include varicella vaccine or vaccines added to the recommended schedule after 1998 for children up to 35 months of age. More information can be found in the Measure Specifications appendix.

Figure 2.21. Composite measure: Children ages 19-35 months who received all recommended vaccines, 2000-2007

- From 2000 to 2007, the percentage of children ages 19-35 months who received all recommended vaccines increased from 72.8% to 80.1% (Figure 2.21).
- Since 2004, the rate has exceeded the Healthy People 2010 target of 80.0%.

Prevention: Children's Dental Care

According to the National Institute of Dental and Craniofacial Research, presence of dental caries is the single most common chronic disease of childhood, occurring five to eight times as frequently as asthma,[22] the second most common chronic disease in children. Regular dental visits help to improve overall oral health and prevent dental caries.

- The percentage of children ages 2-17 with public insurance only who visited a dentist in the calendar year improved from 35.8% in 2002 to 41.4% in 2006 (Figure 2.22). This may, in part, reflect dental services covered by the Children's Health Insurance Program. Rates did not improve significantly overall or for other insurance groups.
- In all data years, uninsured children and children with public insurance only were less likely to visit a dentist in the calendar year than those with any private insurance.

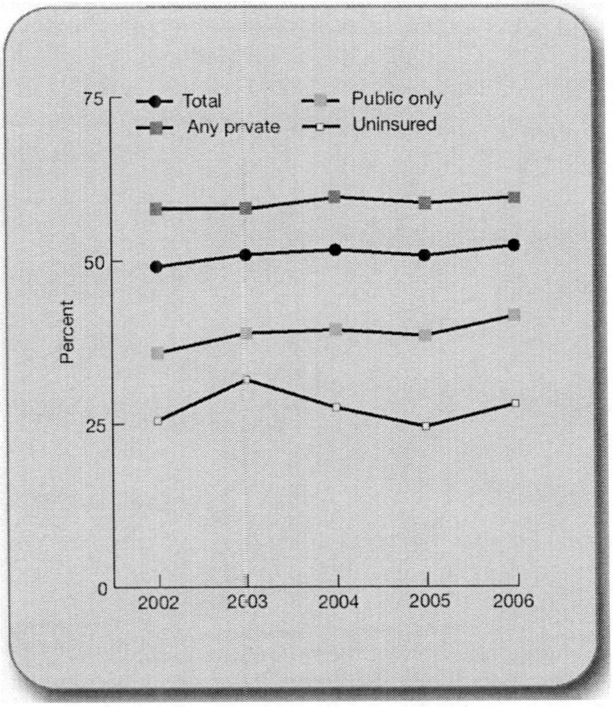

Source: Agency for Healthcare Research and Quality, Medical Expenditure Panel Survey, 2002-2006.
Denominator: U.S. civilian noninstitutionalized population ages 2-17.

Figure 2.22. Children ages 2-17 with a dental visit in the calendar year, by insurance status, 2002-2006

Prevention: Weight Monitoring of Overweight Children

American children are getting heavier. Overweight children are identified using body mass index (BMI) for age growth charts. These growth charts are based on national data collected between 1963 and 1994, and children with BMI values at or above the 95th percentile are considered overweight. From 1976-1980 to 2003-2006, the proportion of children classified as overweight increased from 6.5% to 17% among children ages 6 to 11 and from 5% to 17.6% among adolescents ages 12 to 19.[23] Pediatricians are advised to monitor BMI and excessive weight gain in children in order to recognize and address cases of overweight and obesity.[24] When health care providers alert young patients and their parents about their overweight status, a new opportunity is created to encourage the development of healthy diet and exercise habits that may be carried into adulthood.[24]

- The percentage of people ages 2-19 who were overweight based on height and weight measurement and who were told by a health provider they were overweight did not change significantly between 1999-2002 and 2003-2006 overall or for any age group (Figure 2.23).
- In 2003-2006, overweight children ages 2-5 (22.3%) and 6-11 (35.7%) were less likely than overweight children and teens ages 12-19 (47.5%) to be told by a health provider that they were overweight.

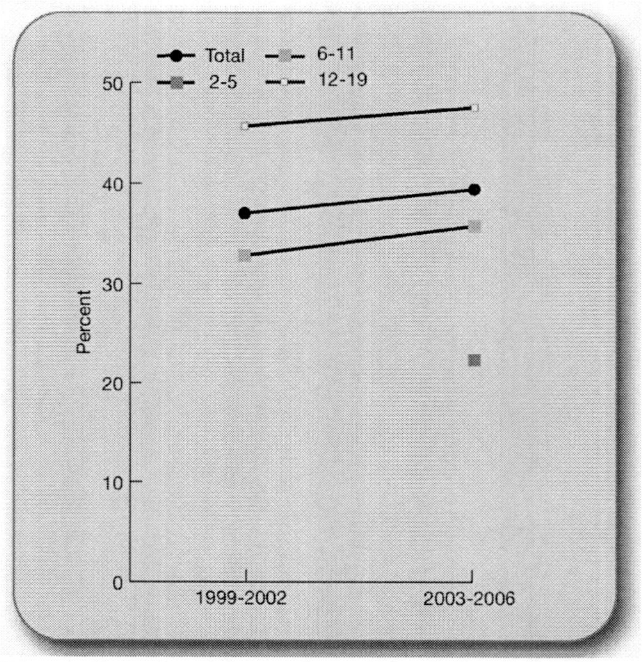

Source: Centers for Disease Control and Prevention, National Center for Health Statistics, National Health and Nutrition Examination Survey, 1999-2002 and 2003-2006.

Denominator: U.S. civilian noninstitutionalized population ages 2-19 who were overweight.

Note: Overweight children are identified using age- and sex-specific reference data from the 2000 Centers for Disease Control and Prevention body mass index (BMI) for age growth charts. Children and youth can be categorized as acceptable, underweight, at risk of overweight, or overweight. Children with BMI values at or above the 95th percentile of the sex-specific BMI growth charts are categorized as overweight. Data for ages 2-5 in 1999-2002 did not meet criteria for statistical reliability.

Figure 2.23. People ages 2-19 who were overweight and who were told by a health provider they were overweight, by age, 1999-2002 and 2003-2006

Prevention: Counseling for Children about Physical Activity

Childhood represents a period when healthy, lifelong habits are often formed. Physicians can play an important role in encouraging healthy behaviors, such as regular exercise, in children.

- From 2002 to 2006, the percentage of children for whom a health provider ever gave advice about the amount and kind of exercise, sports, or physically active hobbies they should have improved from 31.9% to 36.9% (Figure 2.24).
- Between 2002 and 2006, the percentage of children for whom a health provider ever gave advice about physical activity improved for both those with any private insurance and those with only public insurance.
- In all years, uninsured children were less likely than those with any private insurance to have received advice about the amount and kind of exercise, sports, or physically active hobbies they should have.

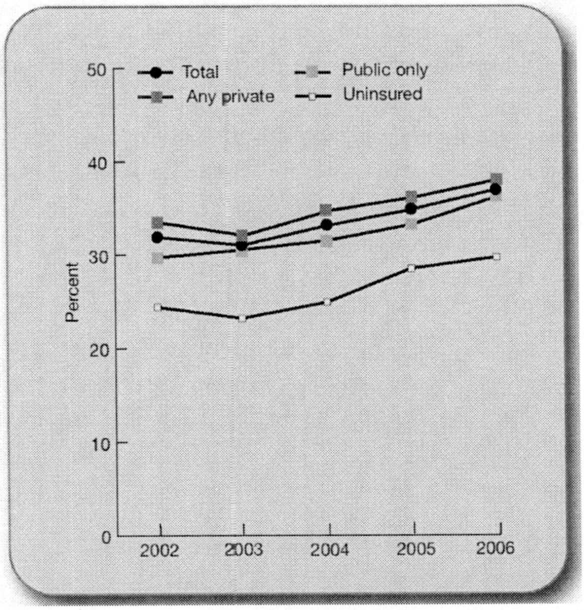

Source: Agency for Healthcare Research and Quality, Medical Expenditure Panel Survey, 2002-2006.
Denominator: U.S. civilian noninstitutionalized population ages 2-17.

Figure 2.24. Children ages 2-17 for whom a health provider ever gave advice about the amount and kind of exercise, sports, or physically active hobbies they should have, by insurance status, 2002-2006

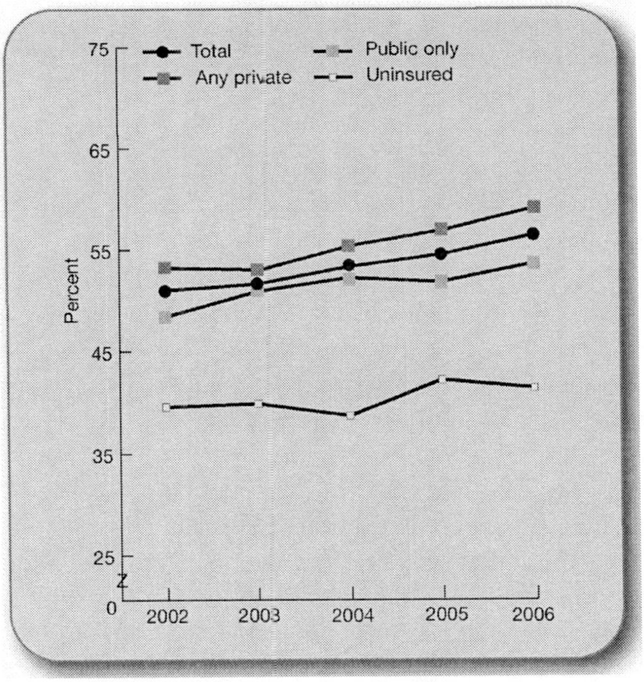

Source: Agency for Healthcare Research and Quality, Medical Expenditure Panel Survey, 2002-2006.
Denominator: U.S. civilian noninstitutionalized population ages 2-17.

Figure 2.25. Children ages 2-17 for whom a health provider ever gave advice about healthy eating, by insurance status, 2002-2006

Prevention: Counseling for Children About Healthy Eating

Physicians play an important role in encouraging children's healthy eating. Overweight and obesity during childhood often persist into adulthood, with consequences that are numerous and costly. Unfortunately, overweight and obesity among children under age 18 have risen dramatically in the past two decades.[24] The American Academy of Pediatrics recommends that pediatricians discuss and promote healthy diets with all children, both those who are overweight and those who are not.[24]

- From 2002 to 2006, the percentage of children for whom a health provider ever gave advice about healthy eating improved from 51.0% to 56.4% (Figure 2.25).
- From 2002 to 2006, the percentage of children for whom a health provider ever gave advice about healthy eating improved for both those with any private insurance and those with only public insurance.
- In all years, uninsured children were less likely to receive advice about healthy eating than those with any private insurance.

Mental Health and Substance Abuse

Importance

Mortality

Number of deaths due to suicide (2006).................... 33,300[2]
Rank among causes of death in the United States—suicide (2006).................. 11th[2]
Alcohol-impaired driving fatalities (2007).. 12,998[25]

Prevalence

People age 12 and over with alcohol and/or illicit drug
dependence or abuse in the past year (2007)...... .... 22.3 million (9.0%)[26]
Adults age 18 and over with serious psychological distress in
the past year (2007) ....24.3 million (10.9%)[26]
Adults age 18 and over with a major depressive episode during
the past year (2007) ....16.5 million (7.5%)[26]
Adults with at least one major depressive episode in their
lifetime (2006)................30.4 million (13.9%)[27]

Cost

National expenditures for the treatment of mental health
and substance abuse disorders (2003 est.)............................ $121 billion[28]
Cost-effectiveness of screening and brief counseling
for problem drinking......................$0-$14,000/QALY[5],[XXIX]

Measures

The NHQR tracks measures of the quality of treatment for major depression and substance abuse. Mental health treatment includes counseling, inpatient care, outpatient care, and prescription medications. This section highlights three core measures of mental health and substance abuse treatment:

- Receipt of treatment for depression.
- Suicide deaths.
- Receipt of needed treatment for illicit drug use or alcohol problem.

In addition, one noncore measure is discussed:

- Completion of substance abuse treatment.

Findings

Treatment: Receipt of Treatment for Depression

Almost 14% of the U.S. population will have a major depressive episode in their lifetime. Treatment can be very effective in reducing symptoms and associated illnesses and returning individuals to a productive lifestyle. For example, the Sequenced Treatment Alternatives to Relieve Depression study provides a blueprint for reasonable medication and psychosocial options for the outpatient management of depression in primary care as well as specialty settings. It showed that by using a measurement-based approach, outcomes in primary care can match those in specialty mental health settings.[29] Ongoing National Institute of Mental Health-funded efforts seek to improve remission rates with existing treatments[30] and to formulate new approaches to treat people with major depression.

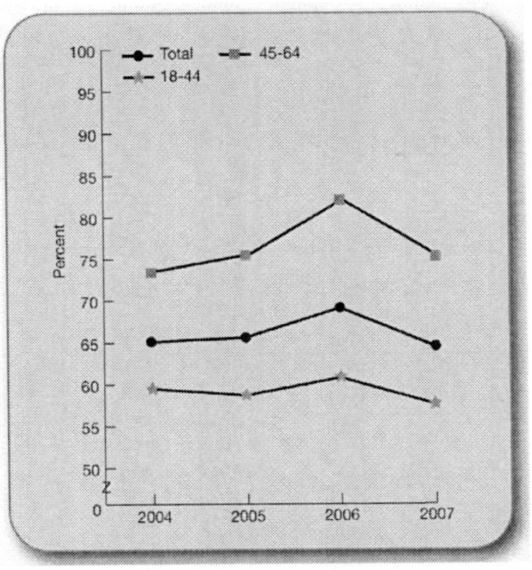

Source: Substance Abuse and Mental Health Services Administration, National Survey on Drug Use and Health, 2004-2007.

Denominator: Adults ages 18-64 with a major depressive episode in the past year.

Note: Total includes adults age 65 and over, but sample sizes are too small to allow separate estimates for this age group.

Figure 2.26. Adults with a major depressive episode in the past year who received treatment for depression in the past year, by age, 2004-2007

- In 2007, 64.5% of adults under age 65 with a major depressive episode received treatment for depression (Figure 2.26). There was no significant improvement in this measure compared with 2004.
- In all years, adults ages 18-44 were less likely to receive treatment for depression than those ages 45-64

Outcome: Suicide Deaths

More than 90% of patients who die by suicide have mental illnesses, such as depression, schizophrenia, or substance abuse.[31] Suicide may be prevented when its warning signs are detected and treated. A previous suicide attempt is among the strongest predictors of subsequent suicide. Cognitive therapy can help those who have attempted suicide consider alternative actions when thoughts of self-harm arise and has been shown to reduce suicide attempts by half during a year of followup.[32]

- Twelve States[XXX] and the District of Columbia were in the best quartile (lowest rates of suicide deaths) in 2006 and had a combined average rate of 8.0 deaths per 100,000 population (Figure 2.27). These States are primarily located in the Northeast.
- The 13 States[XXXI] in the worst quartile (highest rates) in 2006 had a combined average rate of 17.1 deaths per 100,000 population. These States are primarily located in the West.

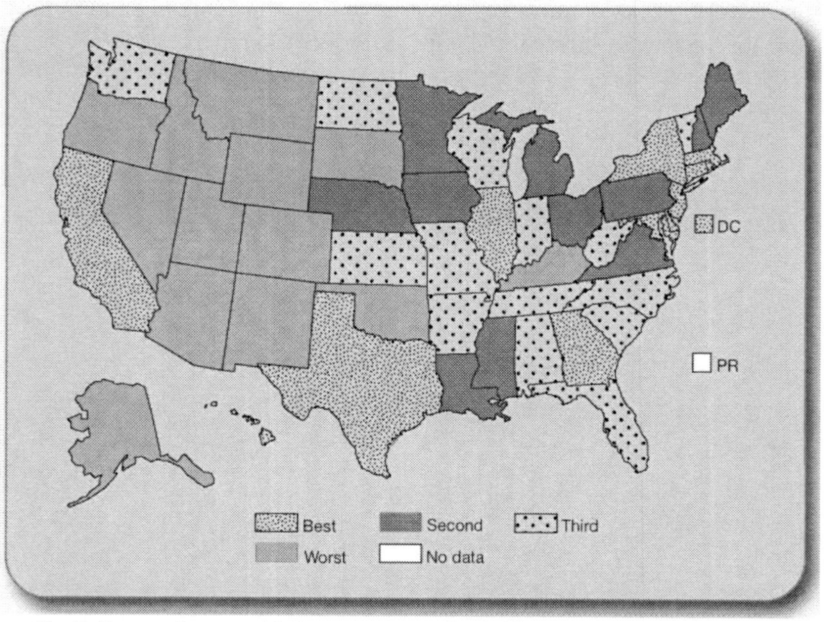

Key: Best quartile indicates States with lowest rates of suicide deaths; worst quartile indicates States with highest rates.

Source: Centers for Disease Control and Prevention, National Center for Health Statistics, National Vital Statistics System—Mortality, 2006.

Denominator: U.S. population.

Note: Rates are age adjusted to the 2000 U.S. standard population.

Figure 2.27. State variation: Suicide deaths per 100,000 population, 2006

Treatment: Receipt of Needed Treatment for Illicit Drug Use or Alcohol Problem

Substance abuse is a medical problem that requires timely treatment, not only because of its health effects but also because drug use is associated with other adverse effects, such as violent behavior. In addition, overall health care costs may be reduced by effective substance abuse and mental health treatment.[33,34] Thus, appropriate receipt and completion of treatment have both clinical and economic implications.

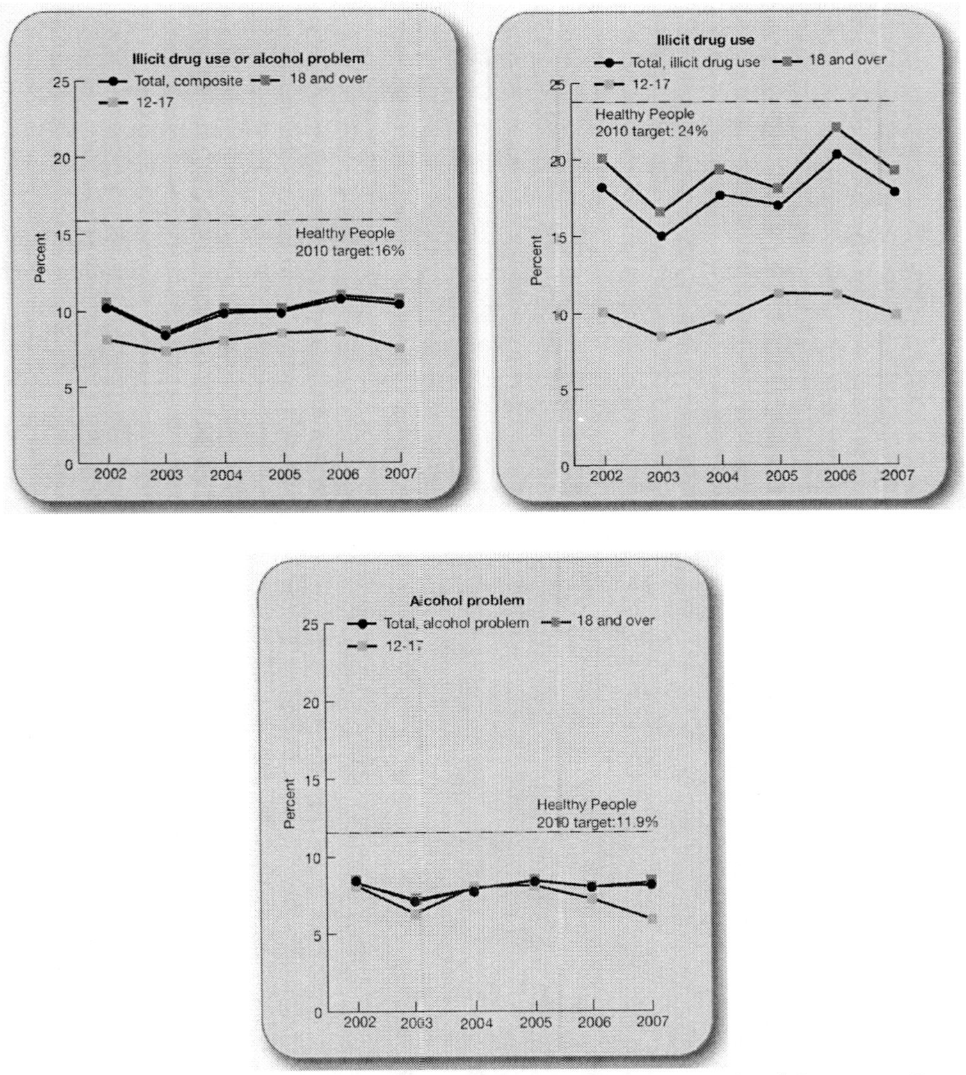

Source: Substance Abuse and Mental Health Services Administration, National Survey on Drug Use and Health, 2002-2007.

Denominator: Civilian noninstitutionalized population age 12 and over who needed treatment for any illicit drug use or alcohol problem.

Note: Treatment refers to treatment at a specialty facility, such as a drug and alcohol inpatient and/or outpatient rehabilitation facility, inpatient hospital setting, or a mental health center.

Figure 2.28. People age 12 and over who needed treatment for illicit drug use or an alcohol problem and who received such treatment at a specialty facility in the last 12 months, overall composite and two components, by age, 2002-2007

- In 2007, 10.4% of people age 12 and over who needed treatment for illicit drug use or an alcohol problem received such treatment. There was no significant change from 2002 to 2007 overall or for any age group (Figure 2.28). For 4 of the 6 data years, adolescents ages 12-17 were significantly less likely to receive treatment for illicit drug use or an alcohol problem compared with adults age 18 and over. As of 2007, the Healthy People 2010 target of 16% had not been met for people who needed treatment and received it for illicit drug use or an alcohol problem.
- Overall, 17.8% of people age 12 and over who met criteria for needing treatment for illicit drug use actually received it in 2007, and this rate has not changed significantly since 2002. In all years, children ages 12-17 who needed treatment for illicit drug use were less likely than adults age 18 and over to receive such treatment. As of 2007, the Healthy People 2010 target of 24% had not been met for people who needed treatment and received it for illicit drug use.
- Overall, 8.1% of people age 12 and over who needed treatment for an alcohol problem received treatment at a specialty facility, and this rate has not changed significantly since 2002. In 2007, adults age 18 and over were more likely than adolescents ages 12-17 to receive treatment for an alcohol problem. As of 2007, the Healthy People 2010 target of 11.9% had not been met for people who needed treatment for an alcohol problem and received it.

Treatment: Completion of Substance Abuse Treatment

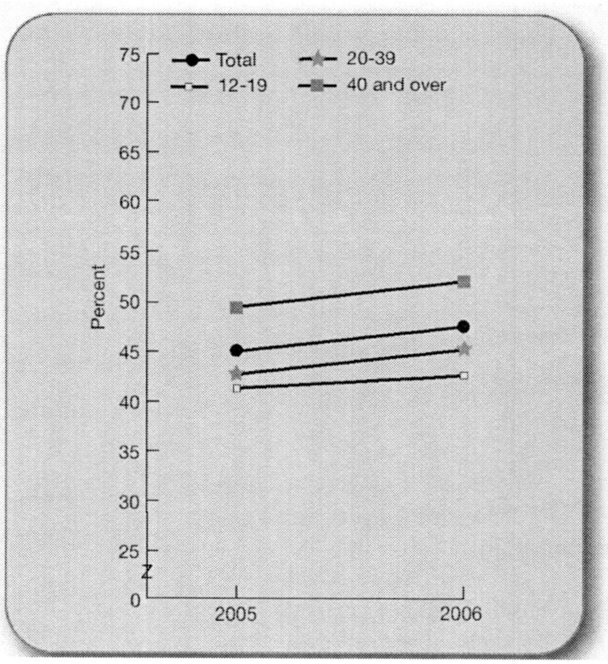

Source: Substance Abuse and Mental Health Services Administration, Treatment Episode Data Set, Discharge Data Set, 2005-2006.

Denominator: Discharges age 12 and over from publicly funded substance abuse treatment facilities.

Figure 2.29. People age 12 and over treated for substance abuse who completed treatment course, by age, 2005-2006

- From 2005 to 2006, the percentage of people age 12 and over treated for substance abuse who completed the treatment course increased from 45.0% to 47.5% (Figure 2.29). A significant increase was also seen for those ages 20-39 and 40 and over.
- In 2006, people ages 12-19 were less likely to complete substance abuse treatment compared with those age 20 and over.

Respiratory Diseases

Importance

Mortality

Number of deaths due to chronic lower respiratory diseases[XXXII] (2006).......... 124,583[2]
Number of deaths, influenza and pneumonia combined (2006)...........56,326[2]
Cause of death rank, chronic lower respiratory diseases (2006)..........4th[2]

Prevalence

Adults age 18 and over who have asthma (2007) .... 16.2 million[35]
Children under age 18 who have asthma (2007)..............6.7 million[36]

Incidence

Annual number of pneumonia cases due to *Streptococcus pneumoniae*........ 500,000[37]
New cases of tuberculosis (2008)........................... 12,898[38]

Cost

Total cost of lung diseases (2009 est.).................$177.4 billion[4]
Direct medical costs of lung diseases (2009 est.) ....$113.6 billion[4]
Total cost of asthma (2007 est.) ....$19.7 billion[39]
Direct medical costs of asthma (2007 est.).....................$14.7 billion[39]
Cost-effectiveness of influenza immunization...................$0-$14,000/QALY[5]

Measures

The NHQR tracks several quality measures for prevention and treatment of this broad category of illnesses that includes influenza, pneumonia, asthma, upper respiratory infection, and tuberculosis. The four core report measures highlighted in this section are:

- Pneumococcal vaccination.
- Receipt of recommended care for pneumonia.
- Completion of tuberculosis therapy.
- Daily asthma medication.

Findings

Prevention: Pneumococcal Vaccination

Vaccination is a cost-effective strategy for reducing illness and death associated with pneumococcal disease of the lungs (pneumonia) and influenza.

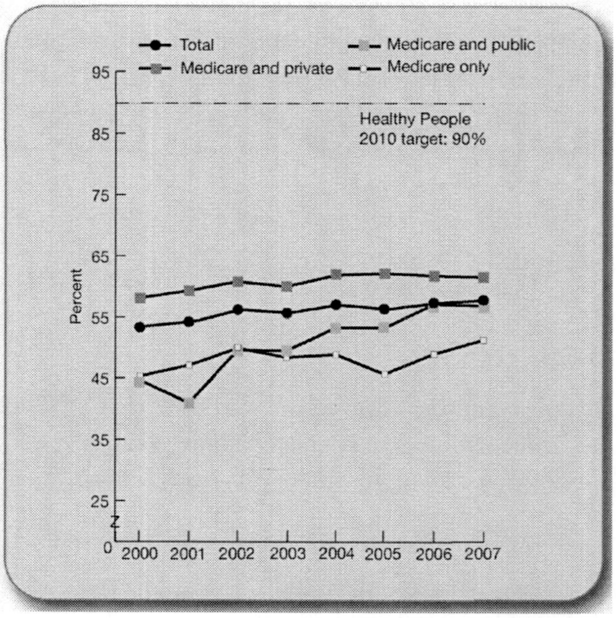

Source: Centers for Disease Control and Prevention, National Center for Health Statistics, National Health Interview Survey, 2000-2007.

Denominator: Civilian noninstitutionalized population age 65 and over.

Note: Age adjusted to the 2000 U.S. standard population.

Figure 2.30. Adults age 65 and over who ever received pneumococcal vaccination, by insurance status, 2000-2007

- The percentage of adults age 65 and over who ever received a pneumococcal vaccination increased from 53.4% in 2000 to 57.8% in 2007 (Figure 2.30). From 2000 to 2007, receipt of pneumococcal vaccination improved for all insurance groups.
- In all years, adults with Medicare only were less likely to receive pneumococcal vaccination compared with adults with Medicare and private insurance. Prior to 2006, adults with Medicare and other public insurance were also less likely to receive pneumococcal vaccination compared with adults with Medicare and private insurance, but these differences were not significant in 2006 or 2007.
- The Healthy People 2010 target of 90% is unlikely to be met at this rate of change.

Treatment: Receipt of Recommended Care for Pneumonia

Recommended care for patients with pneumonia includes receipt of: (1) initial antibiotics within 6 hours of hospital arrival; (2) antibiotics consistent with current recommendations; (3) blood culture before antibiotics are administered; (4) influenza vaccination status assessment/vaccine provision; and (5) pneumococcal vaccination status assessment/vaccine provision. The NHQR tracks receipt of each process measure as well as an overall composite based on an opportunities model. A revision to one measure in 2007 should be noted. The measure of timeliness of initial antibiotic dose was changed from within 4 hours to within 6 hours of hospital arrival. This revised measure is included in the new composite.

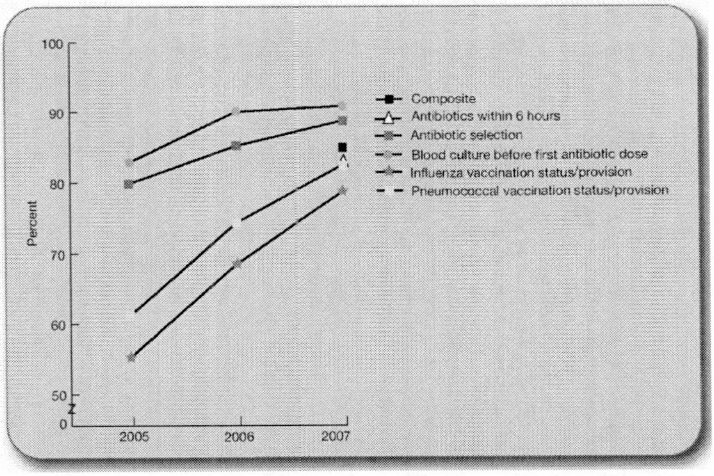

Source: Centers for Medicare & Medicaid Services, Medicare Quality Improvement Organization Program, 2005-2007.

Denominator: Patients hospitalized with a principal discharge diagnosis of pneumonia or a principal discharge diagnosis of either septicemia or respiratory failure and secondary diagnosis of pneumonia.

Note: Data for antibiotics within 6 hours not available for 2005 and 2006.

Figure 2.31. Hospital patients with pneumonia who received recommended hospital care: Overall composite and five components, 2005-2007

- Among the five components of the composite measure, patients were most likely to receive blood cultures before antibiotics (90.8%) and least likely to have their influenza vaccination status assessed (78.7%) (Figure 2.31).
- From 2005 to 2007, rates of appropriate antibiotic selection, blood culture before first antibiotic dose, influenza vaccination, and pneumococcal vaccination all improved.
- The 13 States[XXXIII] in the best quartile (highest rates of receipt of recommended pneumonia care) in 2007 had a combined average rate of 88.8% (Figure 2.32). These States are primarily located in the northern part of the country.
- Eleven States,[XXXIV] the District of Columbia, and Puerto Rico were in the worst quartile (lowest rates) in 2007 and had a combined average rate of 77.5%.

Outcome: Completion of Tuberculosis Therapy

To be effective for individuals as well as the public, tuberculosis therapy must be taken to its completion. Failure to complete tuberculosis therapy puts patients at increased risk for treatment failure and for spreading the disease to others. Even worse, it may result in the development of drug-resistant strains of the disease.[40]

- The percentage of adults ages 18-44 who completed tuberculosis therapy within 1 year increased from 78.2% in 2000 to 82.2% in 2005 (Figure 2.33).
- In all years, children ages 0-17 with tuberculosis were more likely to complete a curative course of treatment within 1 year of treatment than adults age 18 and over.
- Since 2003, the rate among children has exceeded the Healthy People 2010 target of 90%, while rates among other age groups are not on track to meet this target by 2010.

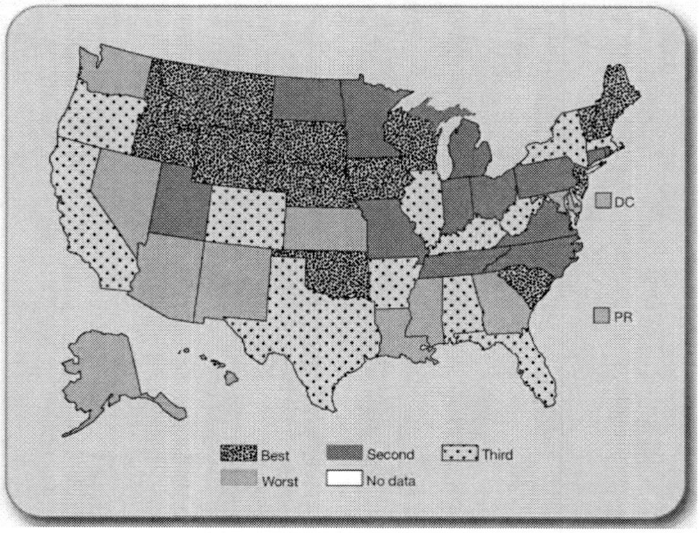

Key: Best quartile indicates States with highest rates of receipt of recommended pneumonia care; worst quartile indicates States with lowest rates.

Source: Centers for Medicare & Medicaid Services, Medicare Quality Improvement Organization Program, 2007.

Denominator: Civilian noninstitutionalized population age 65 and over.

Figure 2.32. State variation: Hospital patients with pneumonia who received recommended hospital care, 2007

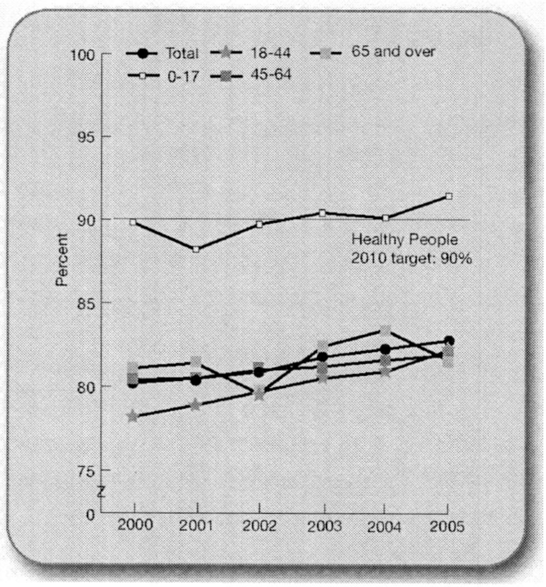

Source: Centers for Disease Control and Prevention, National TB Surveillance System, 2000-2005.

Denominator: U.S. civilian noninstitutionalized population treated for tuberculosis.

Figure 2.33. Patients with tuberculosis who completed a curative course of treatment within 1 year of initiation of treatment, by age, 2000-2005

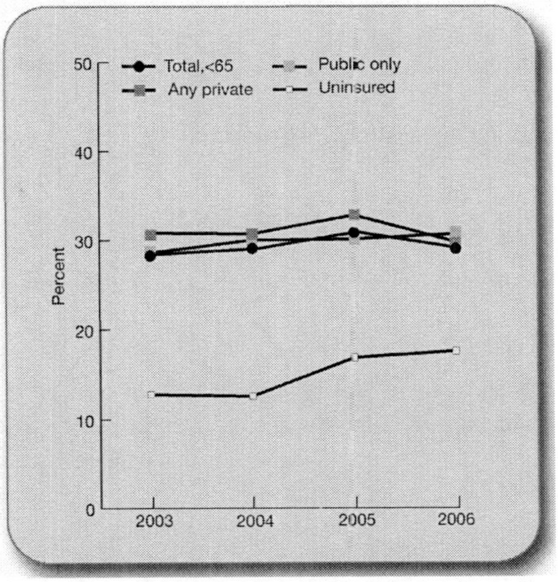

Source: Agency for Healthcare Research and Quality, Medical Expenditure Panel Survey, 2003-2006.
Denominator: Civilian noninstitutionalized population under age 65 who reported current asthma.
Note: People with current asthma report that they still have asthma or had an asthma attack in the last 12 months.

Figure 2.34. People under age 65 with current asthma who are now taking preventive medicine daily or almost daily (either oral or inhaler), by insurance status, 2003-2006

Management: Daily Asthma Medication

Improving quality of care for people with asthma can reduce the occurrence of asthma attacks and avoidable hospitalizations. The National Asthma Education and Prevention Program, coordinated by the National Heart, Lung, and Blood Institute, develops and disseminates science-based guidelines for asthma diagnosis and management.[41] These recommendations are built around four essential components of asthma management critical for effective long-term control of asthma: assessment and monitoring, control of factors contributing to symptom exacerbation, pharmacotherapy, and education for partnership in care.[42]

- Of those with current asthma under age 65 in 2006, 29.1% reported taking preventive medicine daily or almost daily (Figure 2.34).
- In all 4 data years, uninsured people under age 65 with current asthma were less likely than those with private insurance to be taking preventive medicine daily or almost daily.

Lifestyle Modification

Importance

Mortality

Number of deaths per year attributable to smoking (2000-2004) ....443,000[43]

Prevalence

Number of adult current cigarette smokers (2007) .... 43.4 million[44]
Number of obese adults (2005-2006)..................................... >72 million[45]
Number of adults with no leisure-time physical activity (2007) ....84.8 million[35]

Cost

Total cost of smoking (2000-2004 est.) ....$193 billion[43]
Total health care cost related to obesity (2008 est.) ....$147 billion[46]

Measures

Unhealthy behaviors place many Americans at risk for a variety of diseases. Lifestyle practices account for more than 40% of the differences in health among individuals.[47] A recent study examined the effects on incidence of coronary heart disease, stroke, diabetes, and cancer of four healthy lifestyles: never smoking, not being obese, engaging in at least 3.5 hours of physical activity per week, and eating a healthy diet (higher consumption of fruits, vegetables, and whole grain bread and lower consumption of red meat). Engaging in one healthy lifestyle compared with none cut the risk of developing these diseases in half while engaging in all four cut risk by 78%.[48] Unfortunately, healthy lifestyle practices have declined over the past two decades.[48]

Helping patients choose and maintain healthy lifestyles is a critical role of health care. The NHQR tracks several quality measures for modifying unhealthy lifestyles, including the following two core report measures:

- Counseling smokers to quit smoking.
- Counseling obese adults about exercise.

In addition, one noncore measure is presented:

- Counseling obese adults about overweight.

Findings

Prevention: Counseling Smokers to Quit Smoking

Smoking harms nearly every organ of the body and causes or exacerbates many diseases. Smoking causes more than 80% of deaths from lung cancer and more than 90% of deaths from chronic obstructive pulmonary disease.[49] Heart disease is the leading cause of death in the United States for both men and women,[50] with approximately 135,000 deaths due to smoking.[51] Cigarette smoking increases the risk of dying from coronary heart disease (CHD) two- to threefold.[51]

Quitting smoking has immediate and long-term health benefits. The risk of developing CHD attributed to smoking can be decreased by 50% after one year of cessation.[52] Smoking is a modifiable risk factor, and health care providers can help encourage patients to change their behavior and quit smoking.

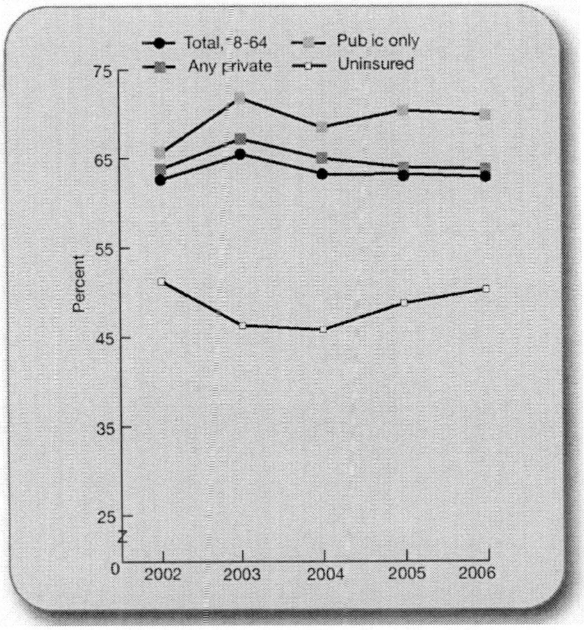

Source: Agency for Healthcare Research and Quality, Medical Expenditure Panel Survey, 2002-2006.
Denominator: Civilian noninstitutionalized adult current smokers under age 65 who had a checkup in the last 12 months.

Figure 2.35. Adult current smokers under age 65 with a checkup in the last 12 months who received advice to quit smoking, by insurance status, 2002-2006

- In 2006, 62.9% of adult current smokers under age 65 with a checkup in the last 12 months received advice to quit smoking (Figure 2.35). From 2002-2006, there were no statistically significant changes overall or for any insurance group in the rates of advice to quit smoking.
- In all years, uninsured adult current smokers under age 65 were less likely to receive advice to quit smoking compared with both privately and publicly insured adult smokers.

Prevention: Counseling Obese Adults About Overweight

More than 34% of adults age 20 and over in the United States are obese (defined as having a BMI of 30 or higher),[45] putting them at increased risk for many chronic, often deadly conditions, such as hypertension, cancer, diabetes, and CHD.[53] Although physician guidelines recommend that health care providers screen all adult patients for obesity,54] obesity remains underdiagnosed among U.S. adults.[55]

- From 1999-2002 to 2003-2006, the total percentage of obese adults age 20 and over who were told by a doctor or health professional they were obese decreased significantly, from 67.8% to 64.8% (Figure 2.36). The decrease among adults ages 45-64 was also significant.
- In both time periods, obese adults ages 20-44 were less likely than those ages 45-64 to be told by a doctor or health professional they were overweight.

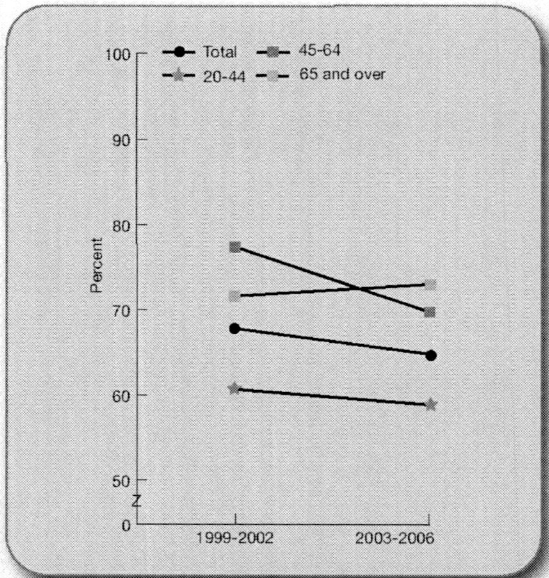

Source: Centers for Disease Control and Prevention, National Center for Health Statistics, National Health and Nutrition Examination Survey, 1999-2002 and 2003-2006.
Denominator: Civilian noninstitutionalized obese adults age 20 and over.

Figure 2.36. Adults with obesity who were told by a doctor they were overweight, by age, 1999-2002 and 2003-2006

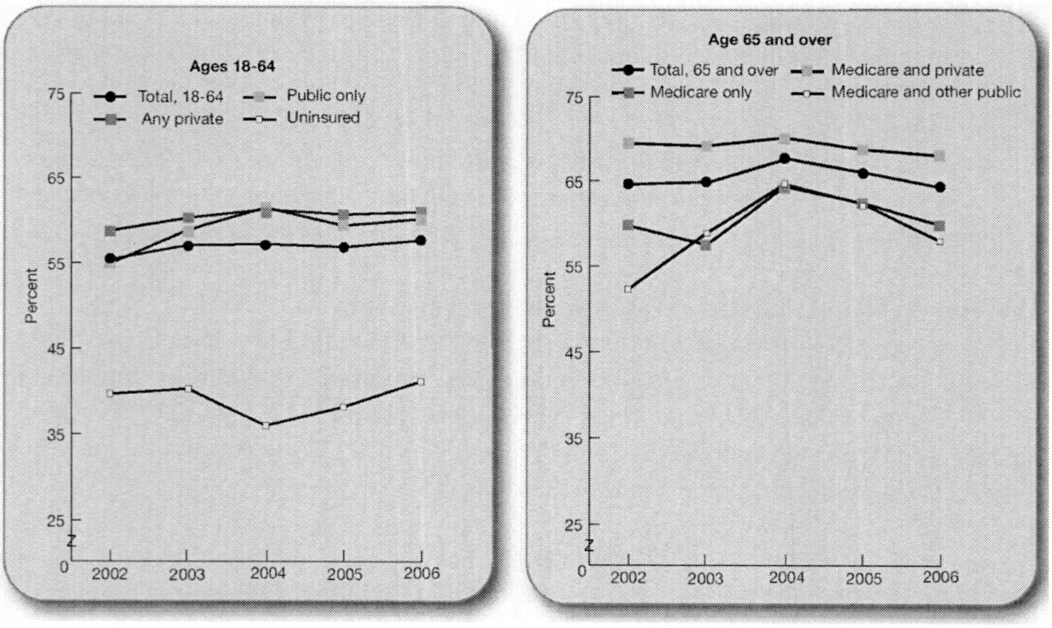

Source: Agency for Healthcare Research and Quality, Medical Expenditure Panel Survey, 2002-2006.
Denominator: Civilian noninstitutionalized adults age 18 and over with obesity.

Figure 2.37. Adults with obesity who ever received advice from a health provider to exercise more, by insurance status, 2002-2006

Prevention: Counseling Obese Adults About Exercise

Physician-based exercise and diet counseling is an important component of effective weight loss interventions,[54] and it has been shown to produce increased levels of physical activity among sedentary patients.[56] Although every obese person may not need counseling about exercise and diet, many would likely benefit from improvements in these activities. Regular exercise and a healthy diet aid in maintaining normal blood cholesterol levels, weight, and blood pressure, reducing the risk of heart disease, stroke, diabetes, and other comorbidities of obesity.

- From 2002 to 2006, rates of advice about exercise did not change overall or for any insurance group (Figure 2.37).
- In all years, among adults under age 65, uninsured individuals were less likely to receive advice about exercise compared with privately or publicly insured individuals.
- Among adults age 65 and over, individuals with Medicare only and Medicare and other public insurance were less likely to receive advice about exercise compared with individuals with Medicare and private insurance in 2002 and 2003, but these differences were not significant in more recent years.

Functional Status Preservation and Rehabilitation

Importance

Demographics

Noninstitutionalized adults needing help of another person with activities of daily living (ADLs)[XXXV] (2007) ....4.4 million[57]

Noninstitutionalized adults age 75 and over needing help of another person with ADLs (2007) ....11%[57]

Noninstitutionalized adults needing help with instrumental activities of daily living (IADLs)[XXXVI] (2007) .... 8.6 million[57]

Noninstitutionalized adults age 75 and over needing help with IADLs (2007)............ 20%[57]

Nursing home residents needing help with ADLs (2004).............................1.5 million[58]

Costs

Medicare payments for outpatient physical therapy (2006 est.)...............$3.1 billion[59]

Medicare payments for outpatient occupational therapy (2006 est.) ....$747 million[59]

Medicare payments for outpatient speech-language pathology services (2006 est.) ....$270 million[59]

Measures

A person's ability to function can decline with disease or age, but it is not always an inevitable consequence. Threats to function span a wide variety of medical conditions. Services to maximize function are delivered in a variety of settings, including providers' offices, patients' homes, long-term care facilities, and hospitals. Some health care interventions can help prevent diseases that commonly cause declines in functional status. Other interventions, such as physical therapy, occupational therapy, and speech-language pathology services, can help patients regain function that has been lost or minimize the rate of decline in functioning.

The NHQR tracks several measures related to functional status preservation and rehabilitation. Three core report measures are highlighted in this section:

- Osteoporosis screening among older women.
- Improvement in ambulation in home health care patients.
- Nursing home residents needing more help with daily activities.

Findings

Prevention: Osteoporosis Screening Among Older Women

Osteoporosis is a disease characterized by loss of bone tissue. About 10 million people in the United States have osteoporosis, and another 34 million with low bone mass are at risk of developing the disease. Women represent more than two-thirds of Americans at risk for or diagnosed with osteoporosis.[60]

Osteoporosis increases the risk of fractures of the hip, spine, and wrist, and about half of all postmenopausal women will experience an osteoporotic fracture. Osteoporotic fractures cost the U.S. health care system $17 billion each year and cause considerable morbidity and mortality. For example, of patients with hip fractures, one-fifth will die during the first year, one-third will require nursing home care, and only one-third will return to the functional status they had before the fracture.[60]

Because older women are at highest risk for osteoporosis, the U.S. Preventive Services Task Force recommends routine osteoporosis screening of women age 65 and over. Women with low bone density can reduce their risk of fracture and subsequent functional impairment by taking appropriate medications.[61]

- From 2001 to 2006, the percentage of older female Medicare beneficiaries who reported ever being screened for osteoporosis with a bone mass or bone density measurement increased overall and among all insurance groups (Figure 2.38).
- In all years, the percentage of older female Medicare beneficiaries who reported ever being screened for osteoporosis was lower among those with Medicare and health maintenance organization, Medicare and Medicaid, or Medicare only compared with those with Medicare and private insurance.

Outcome: Improvement in Ambulation in Home Health Care Patients

After an illness or injury, many patients receiving home health care may need temporary help to walk safely. This assistance can come from another person or from equipment, such as a cane. Patients who use a wheelchair may have difficulty moving around safely, but if they can perform this activity with little assistance, they are more independent, self-confident, and active.

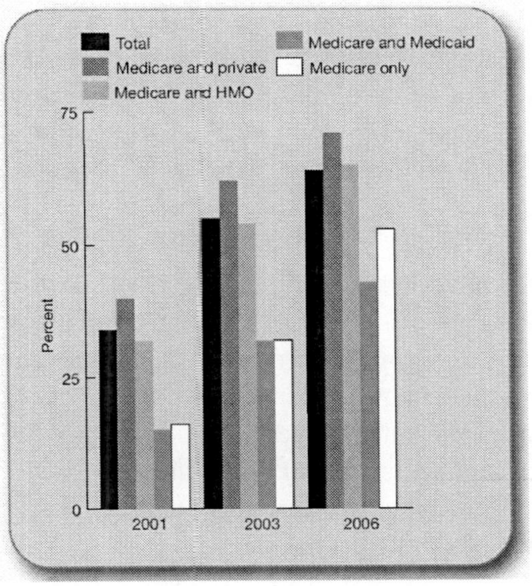

Key: HMO = health maintenance organization
Source: Medicare Current Beneficiary Survey, 2001, 2003, and 2006.
Denominator: Female Medicare beneficiaries age 65 and over living in the community.

Figure 2.38. Older female Medicare beneficiaries who reported ever being screened for osteoporosis with a bone mass or bone density measurement, by insurance status, 2001, 2003, and 2006

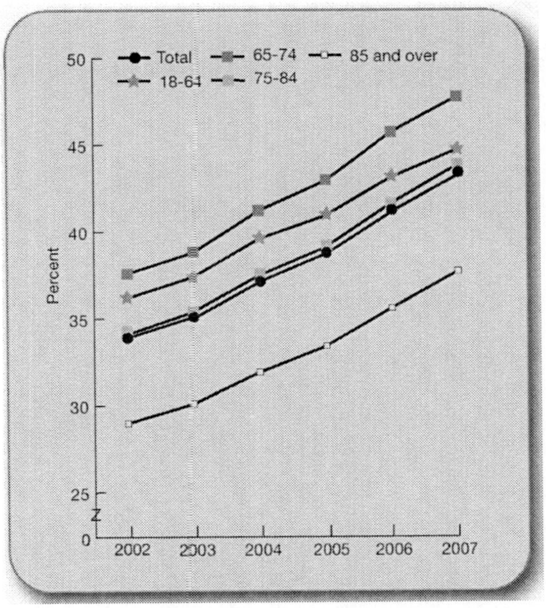

Source: Centers for Medicare & Medicaid Services, Outcome and Assessment Information Set (OASIS), 2002-2007.
Denominator: Adult nonmaternity patients completing an episode of skilled home health care and not already performing at the highest level according to the OASIS question on ambulation at the start of the episode.

Figure 2.39. Adult home health care patients whose ability to walk or move around improved between the start and end of a home health care episode, by age, 2002-2007

As patients recover from illness or injury, many experience improvements in walking and moving with a wheelchair, which can be facilitated by physical therapy. However, in cases of patients with some neurologic conditions, such as progressive multiple sclerosis or Parkinson's disease, ambulation may not improve even when the home health agency provides good care. In addition, the characteristics of patients referred to home health agencies vary across States.

- In 2007, 43.3% of adult home health care patients showed improvement in walking or moving around (Figure 2.39).
- From 2002 to 2007, the percentage of adult home health care patients whose ability to walk or move around improved increased overall and for every age group.
- In all years, home health patients ages 18-64, 75-84, and 85 and over were less likely to show improvement compared with patients ages 65-74. These patients may have higher levels of disability or infirmity than patients ages 65-74 that make improvements in mobility harder to achieve.
- The 13 States[XXXVII] in the best quartile (highest rates of improvement in ability to walk or move around) for home health patients had a combined average rate of 45.6% in 2008 (Figure 2.40). These States are primarily located in the South.

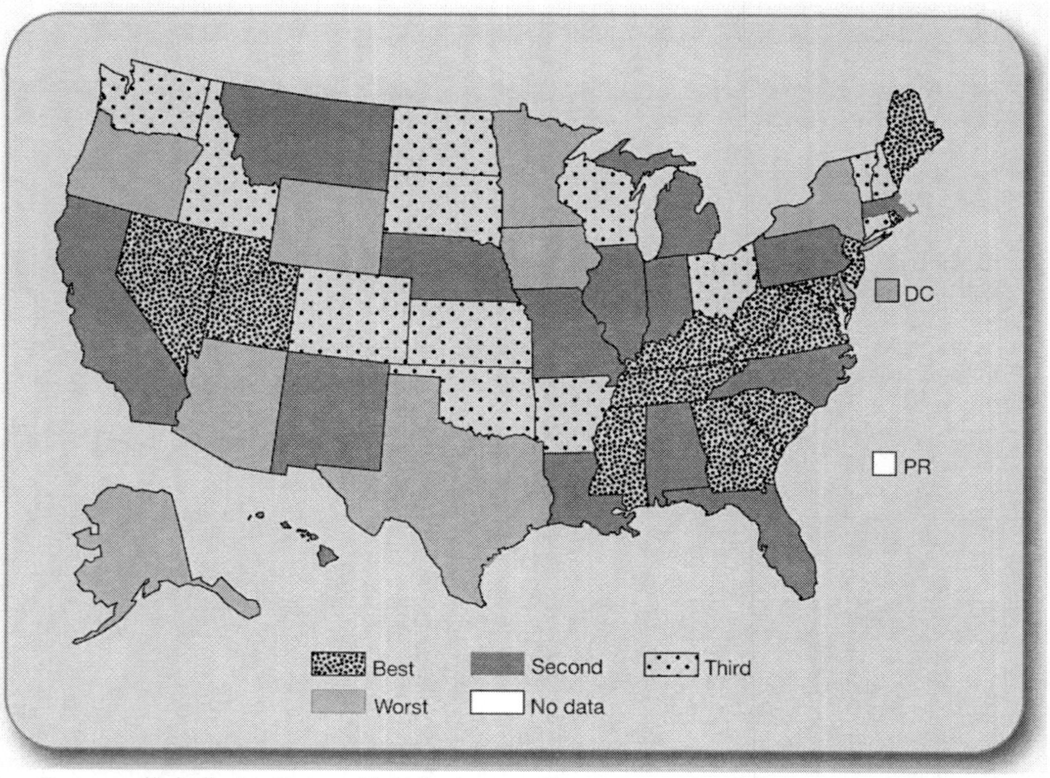

Key: Best quartile indicates States with highest rates of improvement in ability to walk or move around; worst quartile indicates States with lowest rates.

Source: Centers for Medicare & Medicaid Services, Outcome and Assessment Information Set, 2008.

Figure 2.40. State variation: Adult home health care patients whose ability to walk or move around improved, 2008

- Nine States[XXXVIII] and the District of Columbia were in the worst quartile (lowest rates) in 2008, with a combined average rate of 38.7%.

Outcome: Nursing Home Residents Needing More Help with Daily Activities

Patients go to live in nursing homes when they are too frail or sick to be cared for at home. While almost all long-stay nursing home residents have limitations in their activities of daily living, nursing home staff help residents stay as independent as possible. Most residents want to care for themselves, and the ability to perform daily activities is important to their quality of life. Some functional decline among residents cannot be avoided, but optimal nursing home care seeks to minimize the rate of decline.

- The overall percentage of long-stay nursing home residents whose need for help with daily activities increased did not change between 2000 and 2007 (Figure 2.41). The percentage increased among residents ages 0-64 and ages 65-74.
- In all years, residents ages 0-64 were less likely to need increasing help with daily activities compared with residents ages 65-74. In all years except 2007, residents ages 75-84 and age 85 and over were significantly more likely to need increasing help with daily activities compared with residents ages 65-74.

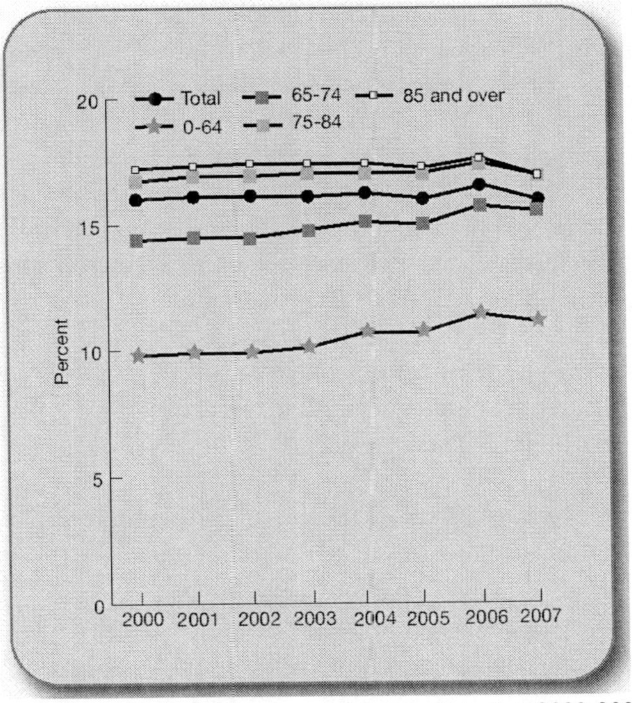

Source: Centers for Medicare & Medicaid Services, Minimum Data Set, 2000-2007. Data are from the third quarter of each calendar year.

Denominator: All long-stay residents in Medicare or Medicaid certified nursing home facilities.

Figure 2.41. Long-stay nursing home residents whose need for help with daily activities increased, by age, 2000-2007

Supportive and Palliative Care

Importance

Demographics

Number of nursing home residents ever admitted during the calendar year (2007)...... .... 3,196,310[62]

Number of Medicare fee-for-service (FFS) home health patients[XXXIX] (2006)......... .... 3,031,814[63]

Number of Medicare FFS beneficiaries using Medicare hospice services (2006)......... ....935,565[64]

Cost

Total costs of nursing home care[XL] (2007 est.)............................$131.3 billion[65]

Total costs of home health care[XL] (2007 est.) ....$59.0 billion[65]

Medicare FFS payments for hospice services (2008 est.) ....11.2 billion[66]

Measures

Disease cannot always be cured, and disability cannot always be reversed. For patients with long-term health conditions, managing symptoms and preventing complications are important goals. Supportive care focuses on enhancing patient comfort and quality of life and preventing and relieving symptoms and complications. Toward the end of life, palliative care also provides patients and families with emotional and spiritual support to help cope with death. Honoring patient values and preferences for care is also critical.[67]

Supportive and palliative care cuts across many medical conditions and is delivered by many health care providers. The NHQR tracks several measures of supportive and palliative care delivered by home health agencies, nursing homes, and hospices. One core report measure on home health care and two core report measures on nursing home care are highlighted in this section:

- Shortness of breath among home health care patients.
- Use of physical restraints on nursing home residents.
- Pressure sores in nursing home residents.

The two noncore measures presented here from the National Hospice and Palliative Care Organization's Family Evaluation of Hospice Care survey are:

- Referral to hospice at the right time.
- Receipt of right amount of pain medicine by hospice patients.

In addition, this NHQR includes a section focusing on pain management from the National Home and Hospice Care Survey.

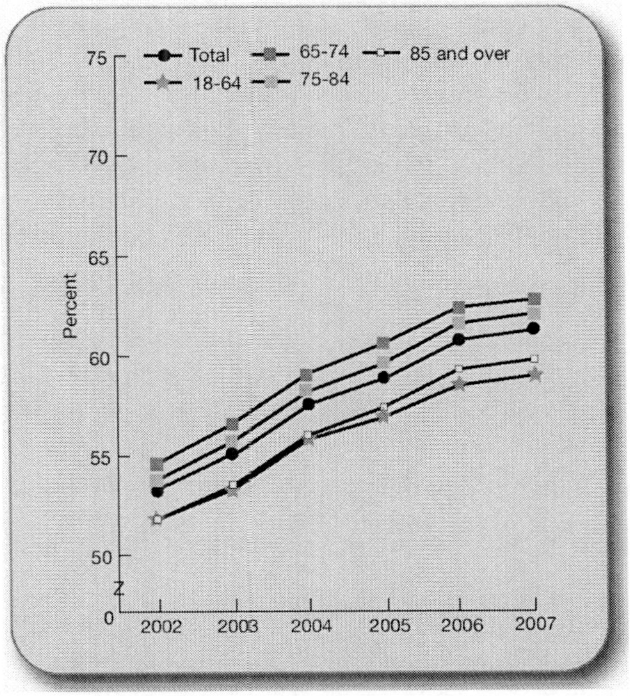

Source: Centers for Medicare & Medicaid Services, Outcome and Assessment Information Set, 2002-2007.

Denominator: Adult nonmaternity patients completing an episode of skilled home health care.

Figure 2.42. Adult home health care patients who had less shortness of breath between the start and end of a home health care episode, by age, 2002-2007

Findings

Outcome: Shortness of Breath among Home Health Care Patients

Shortness of breath is uncomfortable. Many patients with heart or lung problems experience difficulty breathing and may tire easily or be unable to perform daily activities. Doctors and home health staff should monitor shortness of breath and may give advice, therapy, medication, or oxygen to help lessen this symptom.

- Between 2002 and 2007, the percentage of adult home health care patients who had less shortness of breath improved from 53.3% to 61.3% (Figure 2.42). Improvements were observed in all age groups.
- In 2006 and 2007, home health care patients ages 18-64 years were significantly less likely than patients ages 65-74 to have experienced less shortness of breath. Medicare patients under age 65 are usually disabled or have ESRD.

Management: Use of Physical Restraints on Nursing Home Residents

Many medical conditions can cause alterations in mental status. Patients with impaired mental status may fall down, wander, get lost, or become injured. A physical restraint is any device, material, or equipment that keeps a person from moving freely. Some facilities use restraints to prevent some patients from falling or wandering because it is less labor intensive than having staff watch patients closely.

Despite their potential benefits, restraints used daily can lead patients to become weak and develop other medical complications. The use of physical and pharmacologic restraints can result in a variety of emotional, mental, and physical problems. According to regulations for the nursing home industry, restraints should be used only when medically necessary. Bedrails are not included in this measure because they may be appropriate at night for some patients to prevent falls.

- The overall percentage of long-stay nursing home residents who were physically restrained decreased from 10.4% in 2000 to 5.0% in 2007 (Figure 2.43).
- Decreases in the use of physical restraints were observed for all age groups between 2000 and 2007.
- In all years, residents ages 0-64, 75-84, and 85 and over were more likely to be physically restrained compared with residents ages 65-74.

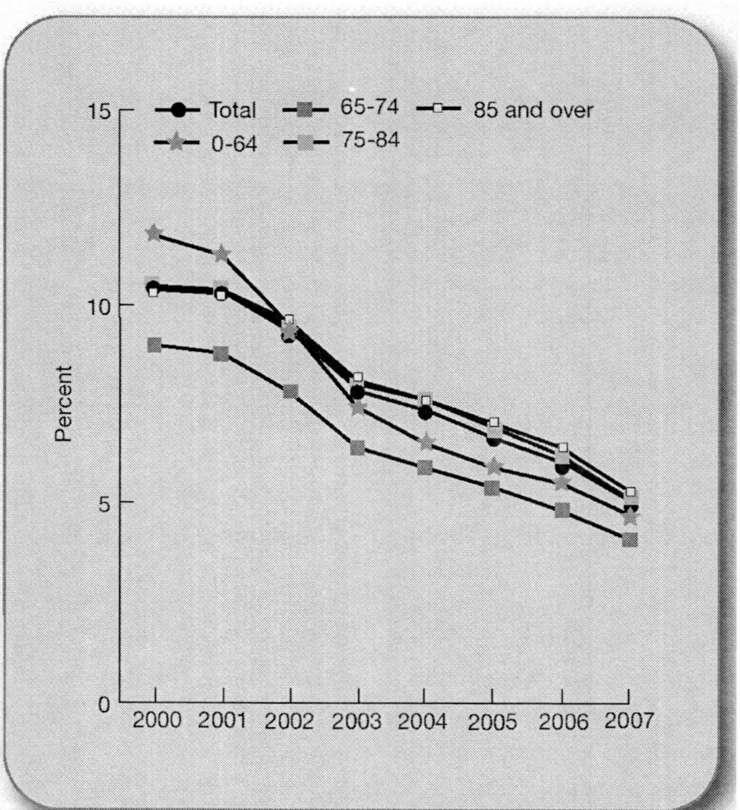

Source: Centers for Medicare & Medicaid Services, Minimum Data Set, 2000-2007. Data are from the third quarter of each calendar year.

Denominator: All long-stay residents in Medicare or Medicaid certified nursing home facilities.

Note: Restraint use was determined based on a 7-day assessment period.

Figure 2.43. Long-stay nursing home residents with physical restraints, by age, 2000-2007

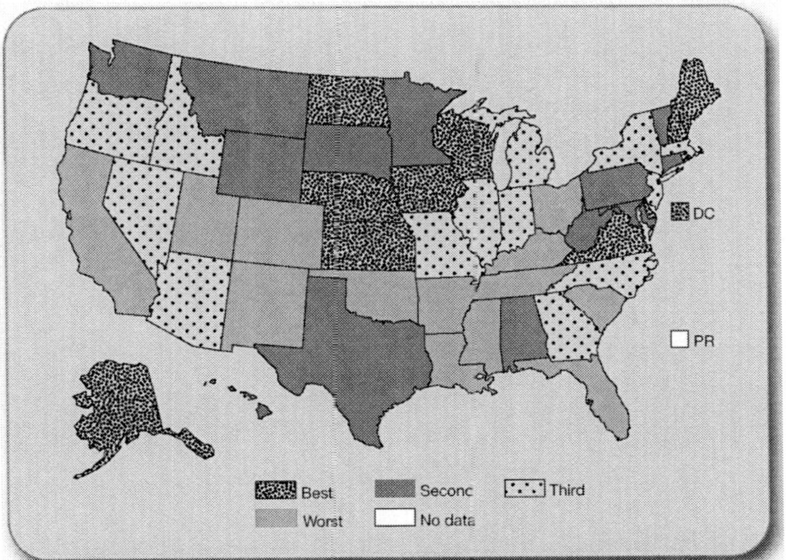

Key: Best quartile indicates States with lowest rates of physical restraints; worst quartile indicates States with highest rates.

Source: Centers for Medicare & Medicaid Services, Minimum Data Set, Nursing Home Compare, 2008.

Figure 2.44. State variation: Long-stay nursing home residents with physical restraints, 2008

- Eleven States[XLI] and the District of Columbia were in the best quartile (lowest rates of physical restraints) in 2008 and had an average rate of 1.4% (Figure 2.44). These States are primarily located in New England and the Midwest.
- The 13 States[XLII] in the worst quartile (highest rates) in 2008 had a combined average rate of 5.9%. These States are primarily located in the South and Southwest.

Outcome: Pressure Sores in Nursing Home Residents

Pressure sores are skin breakdowns caused by sustained sitting or lying in one position for an extended period of time. They can be painful, take a long time to heal, and cause other complications, such as skin or bone infections. Nursing home residents who are bed or chair bound, have difficulty turning and repositioning themselves, are incontinent, and may not receive the nutrients they need to maintain good skin health are at high risk of pressure sores. Residents who lack these characteristics would be considered at low risk of developing pressure sores. Pressure sores require attentive skin care, hygiene, and pressure relief to prevent and heal. The estimates below include pressure sores of all stages.

Nursing home residents differ in their personal care needs and health risks. Short-stay residents commonly have a brief stay in a nursing home after a hospitalization, which is usually followed by return to their home. Long-stay residents, in contrast, are expected to stay in the nursing home either permanently or for an extended time.

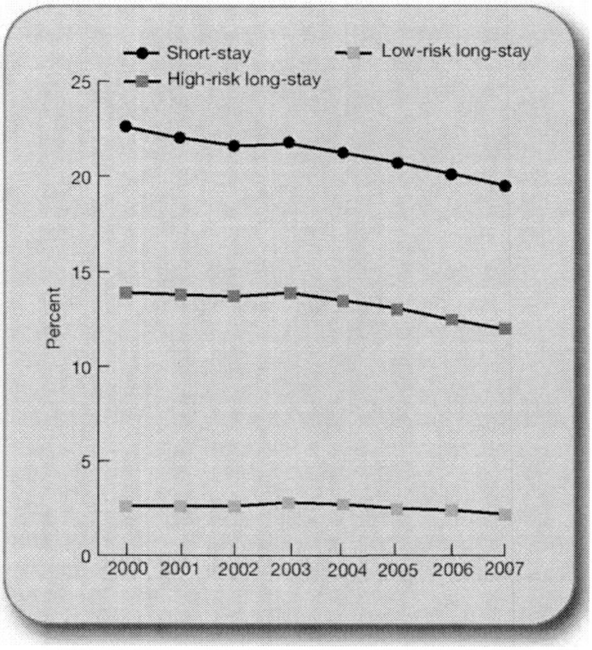

Source: Centers for Medicare & Medicaid Services, Minimum Data Set, 2000-2007.
Denominator: All residents in Medicare or Medicaid certified nursing and long-term care facilities.

Figure 2.45. Short-stay and long-stay nursing home residents with pressure sores, by type of resident, 2000-2007

- From 2000 to 2007, the rate of short-stay residents with pressure sores fell from 22.6% to 19.5% (Figure 2.45).[XLIII] For high-risk long-stay residents, the rate fell from 13.9% to 12.0%, and for low-risk long-stay residents, the rate fell from 2.6% to 2.2%.[XLIV]
- Short-stay residents have the highest rates of pressure sores; some of these patients may be admitted to nursing homes because of sores acquired during an acute care hospitalization. As expected, high-risk long-stay residents have a greater risk of having pressure sores than low-risk long-stay residents.

Management: Referral to Hospice at the Right Time

Hospice care is delivered at the end of life to patients with a terminal illness or condition requiring comprehensive medical care and provides psychosocial and spiritual support for the patient and family. The goal of end-of-life care is to achieve a "good death," defined by the Institute of Medicine as one that is "free from avoidable distress and suffering for patients, families, and caregivers; in general accord with the patients' and families' wishes; and reasonably consistent with clinical, cultural, and ethical standards."[68]

The National Hospice and Palliative Care Organization's Family Evaluation of Hospice Care survey examines the quality of hospice care for dying patients and their family members. Family respondents report how well hospices respect patients' wishes, communicate about illness, control symptoms, support dying on one's own terms, and provide family emotional support.[69],[XLV]

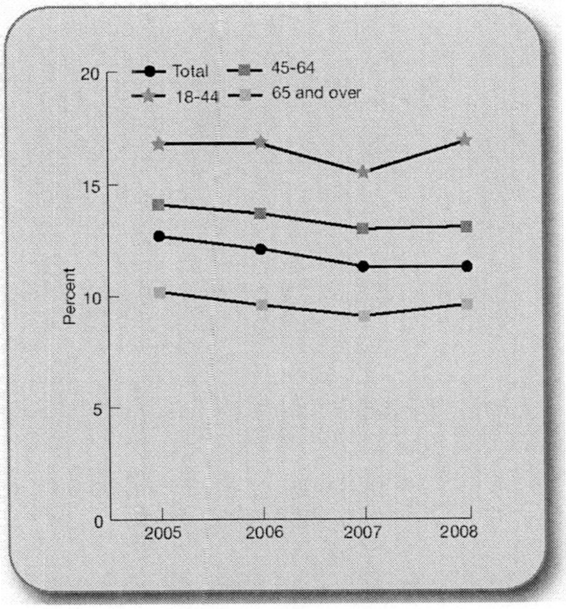

Source: National Hospice and Palliative Care Organization, Family Evaluation of Hospice Care, 2005-2008.

Denominator: Adult hospice patients.

Note: Caregivers were family members who interacted with hospice providers.

Figure 2.46. Hospice patient caregivers who perceived that the patient was NOT referred to hospice at the right time, by age, 2005-2008

Caregivers' perception of the timing of the referral to hospice is often associated with increased reports of unmet needs and lower satisfaction with hospice care. The perception of referral timing may be an indicator of adequacy of access to hospice care.

- The percentage of hospice patient caregivers who perceived that the patient was not referred to hospice at the right time was 11.3% in 2008 (Figure 2.46).
- From 2005 to 2008, caregivers' perception that the patient was referred at the right time improved overall and for patients ages 45-64 and 65 and over.
- In all years, caregivers of patients ages 18-44 and 45-64 were less likely to perceive the patient was referred at the right time compared with caregivers of patients age 65 and over.

Management: Receipt of Right Amount of Pain Medicine by Hospice Patients

Addressing the comfort aspects of care, such as relief from pain, fatigue, and nausea, is an important component of hospice care.[XLVI]

- The percentage of hospice patients whose families reported that they did not receive the right amount of medicine for pain was 5.5% in 2008 (Figure 2.47).
- From 2006 to 2008, the percentage of hospice patients whose families reported that they did not receive the right amount of medicine for pain decreased overall and for adults age 65 and over. There was no significant change during this time period for adults ages 18-44 and ages 45-64.

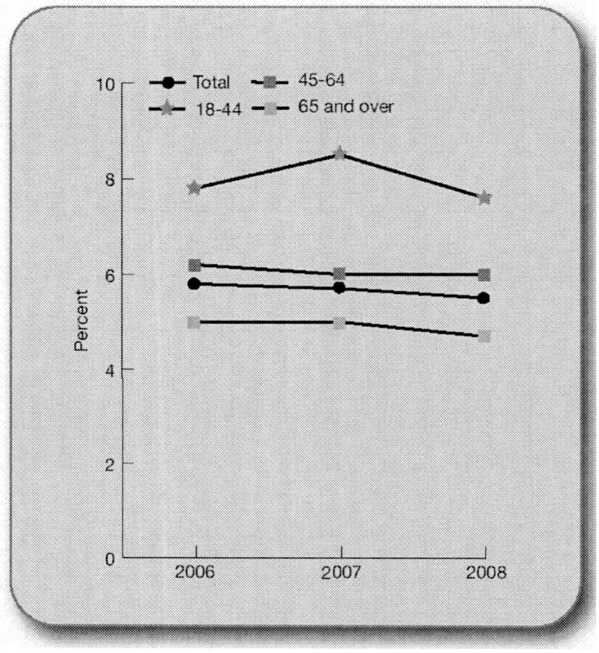

Source: National Hospice and Palliative Care Organization, Family Evaluation of Hospice Care, 2006-2008.

Denominator: Adult hospice patients.

Figure 2.47. Hospice patients who did NOT receive the right amount of medicine for pain, by age, 2006-2008

- In all years, families of hospice patients ages 18-44 and ages 45-64 were more likely to report that the patient did not receive the right amount of pain medicine compared with families of patients age 65 and over.

Focus on Pain Management from the National Home and Hospice Care Survey

Pain management among home health and hospice patients is complex and is made more difficult by the high prevalence of multiple chronic conditions, dementia, and other impairments. Medication only as needed (*pro re nata*, or PRN) is a common pain management strategy. Although appropriate in some cases, this strategy generally yields less than optimal pain control, and high use of PRN-only pain medications may indicate suboptimal management of pain. Administration of medication by standing order is often more clinically appropriate for those with higher pain levels.

This chapter and previous reports have shown the percentage of hospice patients who received the right amount of medicine for pain management based on surveys of families and caregivers. However, information on how pain is managed among home health and hospice patients is generally not available.

The 2007 National Home and Hospice Care Survey (NHHCS) is a nationally representative sample survey of home health and hospice agencies that are either certified by Medicare or Medicaid or licensed by a State to provide home health or hospice services. The total number of agencies that participated in the 2007 NHHCS is 1,036, and data are available on 4,683 current home health patients and 4,733 hospice discharges from these agencies.

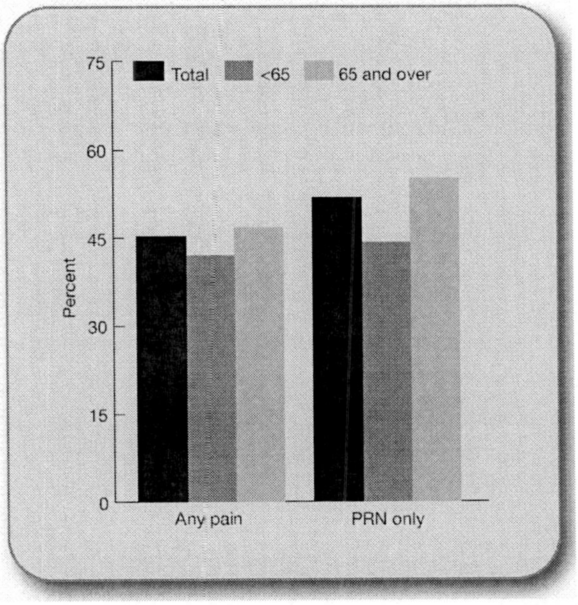

Source: Centers for Disease Control and Prevention, National Center for Health Statistics, National Home and Hospice Care Survey, 2007.

Denominator: Current home health patients.

Figure 2.48. Current home health patients with any pain at last assessment and, if any pain present, only PRN orders for pain management, by age, 2007

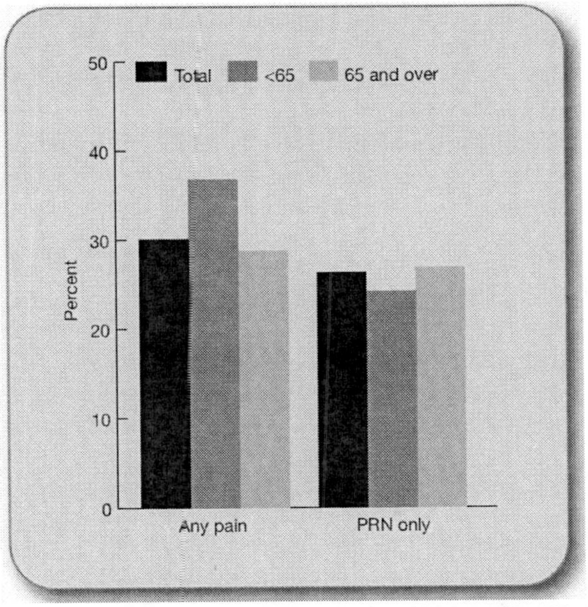

Source: Centers for Disease Control and Prevention, National Center for Health Statistics, National Home and Hospice Care Survey, 2007.

Denominator: Hospice care discharges with pain assessment.

Figure 2.49. Hospice care discharges with any pain at last assessment and, if any pain present, only PRN orders for pain management, by age, 2007

The 2007 NHHCS data were collected through in-person interviews with agency directors and their designated staff; no interviews were conducted directly with patients or their families and friends. NHHCS also collected information from patient records on the occurrence, intensity, and management of pain. Separate analyses of pain management of home health patients and hospice care discharges are presented.

- Among current home health patients, 45.3% were assessed to have any pain at the last assessment (Figure 2.48).
- Of current home health patients with any pain, 51.9% were managed with PRN orders only. Differences by age were not statistically significant.
- Among hospice care discharges in 2007, 30.1% of assessed patients had pain at the last assessment (Figure 2.49).
- Of hospice care discharges in which the patient had any pain, 26.3% were managed with PRN orders only.
- Hospice care discharges of patients under age 65 were more likely to have any pain at last assessment compared with hospice discharges of patients age 65 and over, but management of pain with PRN orders only was similar between the two age groups.

References

[1] American Cancer Society. Cancer facts and figures 2009. Atlanta, GA: American Cancer Society; 2009. Available at: http://www.cancer.org/docroot/STT/STT_0.asp. Accessed on May 7, 2009.

[2] Heron, M; Hoyert, D; Murphy, S. et al. Deaths: Final data for 2006. *National Vital Statistics Reports,* 2009, 57(14).

[3] Surveillance Epidemiology and End Results (SEER) Program. *Prevalence database: U.S. estimates complete prevalence counts on 1/1/2005*. Bethesda, MD: National Cancer Institute, Division of Cancer Control and Population Sciences, Surveillance Research Program, Statistical Research and Applications Branch; 2008. Released April 2008, based on November 2007 SEER data submission.

[4] National Heart, Lung, and Blood Institute. Fact book fiscal year 2008. Bethesda, MD: National Institutes of Health; 2008. Available at: http://www.nhlbi.nih.gov/about/factpdf.htm. Accessed on May 7, 2009.

[5] Maciosek, MV; Coffield, AB; Edwards, NM. et al. Priorities among effective clinical preventive services: results of a systematic review and analysis. *Am J Prev Med,* 2006 Jul, 31(1), 52-61.

[6] U.S. Department of Health and Human Services. Healthy People 2010. Washington, D.C.: U.S. Government Printing Office; 2000. Available at: http://www.healthypeople.gov/. Accessed on March 18, 2009.

[7] U.S. Preventive Services Task Force. Screening for breast cancer: recommendations and rationale. In: Guide to clinical preventive services, 2d ed. Available at: http://www.ahrq.gov/clinic/uspstf/uspsbrca.htm. Accessed on March 19, 2009.

[8] National diabetes fact sheet. Atlanta: Centers for Disease Control and Prevention; 2008. Available at: http://www.cdc.gov/diabetes/pubs/estimates07.htm. Accessed on June 30, 2008.

[9] National Center for Chronic Disease Prevention and Health Promotion. Diabetes: successes and opportunities for population-based prevention and control: at a glance 2009. Atlanta: Centers for Disease Control and Prevention; 2009. Available at: http://www.cdc.gov/nccdphp/publications/aag/pdf/diabetes.pdf. Accessed on November 14, 2008.

[10] U.S. Renal Data System. USRDS 2008 annual data report: atlas of chronic kidney disease and end-stage renal disease in the United States. Bethesda, MD: National Institutes of Health, National Institute of Diabetes and Digestive and Kidney Diseases; 2008. Available at: http://www.usrds.org/atlas.htm. Accessed on February 23, 2009.

[11] U.S. Renal Data System. USRDS 2009 annual data report: atlas of chronic kidney disease and end-stage renal disease in the United States. Bethesda, MD: National Institutes of Health, National Institute of Diabetes and Digestive and Kidney Diseases; 2009. Available at: http://www.usrds.org/adr.htm. Accessed on December 22, 2009.

[12] Healthcare Systems Bureau. Division of Transplantation. 2007 annual report of the U.S. Organ Procurement and Transplantation Network and Scientific Registry of Transplant Recipients: transplant data 1997-2006. Rockville, MD: Health Resources and Services Administration; 2007. Available at: http://optn.transplant.hrsa.gov/data/annual Report.asp. Accessed on November 3, 2008.

[13] American Heart Association. Heart disease and stroke statistics — 2009 update. Dallas, TX: American Heart Association; 2009. Available at: http://www. americanheart.org/presenter.jhtml?identifier=1200026. Accessed on March 25, 2009.

[14] Rosamond, W; Flegal, K & Friday, G. et al. Heart disease and stroke statistics—2007 update: a report from the American Heart Association Statistics Committee and Stroke Statistics Subcommittee. *Circulation,* 2007 Feb 5, 115(5), e69-171.

[15] HIV/AIDS Surveillance Report. 2007. Vol. 19. Atlanta: Centers for Disease Control and Prevention; 2009. Available at: http://www.cdc.gov/hiv/ topics/surveillance/resources/reports/2007report/pdf/2007SurveillanceReport.pdf. Accessed on March 27, 2009.

[16] U.S. Federal funding for HIV/AIDS: The President's FY 2010 budget request; 2009. Menlo Park, CA: The Henry J. Kaiser Family Foundation; 2009. Available at: http://www.kff.org/hivaids/upload/7029-05.pdf. Accessed on December 22, 2009.

[17] Centers for Disease Control and Prevention. HIV/AIDS Surveillance Report, 2007. Vol. 19, Table 8. Atlanta: U.S. Department of Health and Human Services, Centers for Disease Control and Prevention; 2009. Available at: http://www.cdc.gov/hiv/topics/surveillance/ resources/reports/2007report/table8.htm.

[18] Opportunistic infection prophylaxis. In: Clinical management of the HIV-infected adult. Newark, NJ: AIDS Education & Training Centers National Resource Center; 2006. p. 2-35-2-38. Available at: http://www.aidsetc.org/aidsetc?page=cm-207_oipx. Accessed on May 6, 2007.

[19] 2007 American Community Survey 1-year estimates, Table S0901, children characteristics; 2007. Suitland, MD: U.S. Census Bureau; 2007. Available at: http://factfinder.census.gov/servlet/STTable?_bm=y&-qr_name=ACS_2007_1YR_G00_S0901&-geo_id=01000US&-

ds_name=ACS_2007_1YR_G00_&-_lang=en&-redoLog=false. Accessed on March 10, 2009.

[20] Martin, JA; Hamilton, BE; Sutton. PD. et al. Births: final data for 2006. *National Vital Statistics Reports* 2009, 57(7), Available at: www.cdc.gov/nchs/data/nvsr/nvsr57/ nvsr57_07.pdf. Accessed on March 10, 2009.

[21] Total health services—mean and median expenses per person with expense and distribution of expenses by source of payment: United States, 2002. Medical Expenditure Panel Survey component data. Rockville, MD: Agency for Healthcare Research and Quality; 2005.

[22] U.S. Department of Health and Human Services. Oral health in America: a report of the Surgeon General. Rockville, MD: U.S. Department of Health and Human Services, National Institutes of Health, National Institute of Dental and Craniofacial Research; 2000. Available at: http://www.surgeongeneral.gov/library/oralhealth/. Accessed on December 19, 2007.

[23] Ogden, CL; Carroll, MD; Flegal, KM. High body mass index for age among U.S. children and adolescents, 2003-2006. *JAMA*. 2008, 299(20), 2401-5.

[24] Krebs, NF; Jacobson, MS. Prevention of pediatric overweight and obesity. *Pediatrics,* 2003 Aug, 112(2), 424-30.

[25] National Highway Traffic Safety Administration, National Center for Statistics and Analysis. 2007 traffic safety annual assessment—alcohol-related fatalities. Traffic Safety Facts Research Note. Washington, DC: U.S. Department of Transportation; 2008. Publication No. DOT HS 811 016. Available at: http://www-nrd.nhtsa.dot.gov/Pubs/811016.PDF. Accessed on April 6, 2009.

[26] Substance Abuse and Mental Health Services Administration. Results from the 2007 National Survey on Drug Use and Health: national findings. Rockville, MD: Office of Applied Studies; 2008. NSDUH Series H-34. Publication No. SMA 08-4343. Available at: www.oas.samhsa.gov/nsduh/2k7nsduh/2k7results.pdf. Accessed on April 6, 2009.

[27] Substance Abuse and Mental Health Services Administration. Results from the 2006 National Survey on Drug Use and Health: national findings. Rockville, MD: Office of Applied Studies; 2007. NSDUH Series H-32. Publication No. 07-4293. Rockville, MD: Office of Applied Studies; 2006. Available at: www.oas.samhsa.gov /nsduh/2k6nsduh/2k6results.pdf. Accessed on March 27, 2008.

[28] Mark, T; Levit, K; Coffey, R. et al. National expenditures for mental health services and substance abuse treatment, 1993-2003. Rockville, MD: Substance Abuse and Mental Health Services Administration; 2007. Publication No. SMA 07-4227. Available at: http://www.samhsa.gov/ spendingestimates/SAMHSAFINAL9303.pdf. Accessed on November 14, 2008.

[29] Gaynes, BN; Rush, AJ; Trivedi, MH. et al. Primary versus specialty care outcomes for depressed outpatients managed with measurement-based care: results from STAR*D. *J Gen Intern Med,* 2008 May, 23(5), 551-60.

[30] Insel, TR; Wang, PS. The STAR*D trial: revealing the need for better treatments. *Psychiatr Serv,* 2009 Nov, 60(11), 1466-7.

[31] Moscicki E. Epidemiology of completed and attempted suicide: toward a framework for prevention. *Clin Neurosci Res,* 2001, 1, 310-23.

[32] Brown, GK, Ten Have, T; Henriques, GR. et al. Cognitive therapy for the prevention of suicide attempts: a randomized controlled trial. *JAMA,* 2005 Aug 3; 94(5), 563-70.

[33] Lave J. The cost offset effect. *Mental health policy for older Americans: protecting minds at risk.* Washington, DC: American Psychiatric Press; 1990.

[34] Luchansky, B; Longhi, D. Briefing paper: cost savings in Medicaid medical expenses: an outcome of publicly funded chemical dependency treatment in Washington State. Olympia: Washington State Department of Social and Health Services; 1997. No. 4.29. Available at: http://www1.dshs.wa.gov/pdf/ms/rda/research/4/30.pdf. Accessed on November 14, 2008.

[35] Pleis, JR; Lucas, JW. Summary health statistics for U.S. adults: National Health Interview Survey, 2007. National Center for Health Statistics. *Vital Health Stat,* 2009, 10(240).

[36] Bloom, B; Cohen, RA. Summary health statistics for U.S. children: National Health Interview Survey, 2007. National Center for Health Statistics. *Vital Health Stat,* 2009, 10(239).

[37] National Institutes of Health, National Institute of Allergy and Infectious Diseases, Office of Communications and Public Liaison. Pneumococcal pneumonia: cause; 2004. Available at: http://www3.niaid.nih.gov/topics/pneumonia/Cause.htm.Accessed on November 14, 2008.

[38] Centers for Disease Control and Prevention. Trends in tuberculosis Incidence—United States, 2008. MMWR 2009;58(10):249-53.

[39] National Heart, Lung, and Blood Institute. Morbidity and mortality. 2007 chart book on cardiovascular, lung, and blood diseases. Bethesda, MD: National Institutes of Health; 2007. Available at: http://www.nhlbi.nih.gov/resources/docs/07a-chtbk.pdf. Accessed on June 18, 2008.

[40] National Institute of Allergy and Infectious Diseases. Tuberculosis. Bethesda, MD: National Institutes of Health; 2006. Available at: http://www3.niaid.nih.gov/topics/tuberculosis. Accessed on November 14, 2008.

[41] National Heart, Lung, and Blood Institute, National Asthma Education and Prevention Program. Expert Panel Report 3: guidelines for the diagnosis and management of asthma. Full report 2007. Bethesda MD: National Institutes of Health; 2007. Publication No. NIH 07-4051. Available at: http://www.nhlbi.nih.gov/guidelines/asthma/asthgdln.pdf. Accessed on November 4, 2008.

[42] National Heart, Lung, and Blood Institute. National Asthma Education and Prevention Program. Key clinical activities for quality asthma care: recommendations of the National Asthma Education and Prevention Program. *MMWR,* 2003, 52(RR06), 1-8. Available at: http://www.cdc.gov/mmwr/preview/mmwrhtml/rr5206a1.htm.

[43] Centers for Disease Control and Prevention. Smoking-attributable mortality, years of potential life lost, and productivity losses—United States, 2000—2004. *MMWR* 2008, 57(45), 1226-8.

[44] Centers for Disease Control and Prevention. Cigarette smoking among adults—United States, 2007. *MMWR,* 2008 November, 57(45), 1221-6.

[45] Ogden, CL; Carroll, MD; McDowell, MA. et al. *Obesity among adults in the United States—no statistically significant change since 2003–2004.* NCHS Data Brief No. 1. Hyattsville, MD: National Center for Health Statistics; 2007. Available at: www.cdc.gov/nchs/data/databriefs/db01.pdf. Accessed on June 1, 2009.

[46] Finkelstein, EA; Trogdon, JG; Cohen, JW. et al. Annual medical spending attributable to obesity: payer- and service-specific estimates. *Health Aff (Millwood),* 2009 Sep-Oct, 28(5), w822-31. Epub 2009 Jul 27.

[47] Satcher, D; Higginbotham, EJ. The public health approach to eliminating disparities in health. *Am J Public Health,* 2008 Sep, 98(9 Suppl), S8-11.

[48] Ford, ES; Bergmann, MM; Kroger, J. et al. Healthy living is the best revenge: findings from the European Prospective Investigation Into Cancer and Nutrition-Potsdam study. *Arch Intern Med,* 2009 Aug 10, 169(15), 1355-62.

[49] The health consequences of smoking: a report of the Surgeon General. Atlanta: U.S. Department of Health and Human Services, Centers for Disease Control and Prevention, National Center for Chronic Disease Prevention and Health Promotion, Office on Smoking and Health; Washington, DC: Government Printing Office; 2004. Available at: http://www.cdc.gov/tobacco/data_statistics/sgr/2004/index.htm

[50] Hoyert, D; Kung, H; Smith, B. Deaths: preliminary data for 2003. *National Vital Statistics Reports* 2005, 53(15), Available at: www.cdc.gov/ nchs/data/nvsr /nvsr53/nvsr53_15.pdf. Accessed on November 13, 2008.

[51] Cigarette smoking and cardiovascular diseases. Dallas, TX: American Heart Association; 2008. Available at: http://www.americanheart. org/presenter.jhtml ?identifier=4545. Accessed on August 12, 2009.

[52] U.S. Department of Health and Human Services. The health benefits of smoking cessation: a report of the Surgeon General. Rockville, MD: U.S. Department of Health and Human Services, Centers for Disease Control and Prevention, National Center for Chronic Disease Prevention and Health Promotion, Office on Smoking and Health; Washington, DC: Government Printing Office; 1990. Publication No. CDC 90-8416. Available at: http://profiles.nlm.nih.gov/NN/B/B/C/T/_/nnbbct.pdf. Accessed on November 14, 2008.

[53] Centers for Disease Control and Prevention, National Center for Chronic Disease Prevention and Health Promotion, Division of Nutrition and Physician Activity. Overweight and obesity. Atlanta; 2008. Available at: http://www.cdc.gov/ nccdphp/dnpa/obesity/. Accessed on May 8, 2006.

[54] U.S. Preventive Services Task Force. *Screening for obesity in adults: recommendations and rationale*. Rockville, MD: Agency for Healthcare Research and Quality; 2003. Available at: http://www.ahrq.gov/clinic/3rduspstf/obesity/obesrr.htm. Accessed on May 8, 2008.

[55] Diaz, VA; Mainous, AG; 3rd, Koopman, RJ. et al. Undiagnosed obesity: implications for undiagnosed hypertension, diabetes, and hypercholesterolemia. *Fam Med,* 2004 Oct, 36(9), 639-44.

[56] Calfas, KJ; Long, BJ; Sallis, JF. et al. A controlled trial of physician counseling to promote the adoption of physical activity. *Prev Med* ,1996 May-Jun, 25(3), 225-33.

[57] Adams, PF; Barnes, PM; Vickerie, JL. Summary health statistics for the U.S. population: National Health Interview Survey, 2007. National Center for Health Statistics. *Vital Health Stat,* 2008, 10(238).

[58] National Center for Health Statistics, Division of Health Care Statistics. 2004 National Nursing Home Survey. Hyattsville, MD: Centers for Disease Control and Prevention.

[59] Ciolek, D; Hwang, W. CY 2006 outpatient therapy services utilization report. Baltimore, MD: Prepared for Centers for Medicare & Medicaid Services; 2008.

Availableat:www.cms.hhs.gov/TherapyServices/downloads/2_CY2006Outpatient TherapyUtilization Report_PDF_Final.pdf. Accessed on August 12, 2009.
[60] Lane, NE. Epidemiology, etiology, and diagnosis of osteoporosis. *Am J Obstet Gynecol,* 2006 Feb, 194(2 Suppl), S3-11.
[61] U.S. Preventive Services Task Force. Screening for osteoporosis in postmenopausal women: recommendations and rationale. In: Guide to clinical preventive services, 3d ed. Available at: www.ncbi.nlm.nih.gov/bookshelf/br.fcgi?book=hscps3 edrec&part=A 289. Accessed on August 12, 2009.
[62] Nursing home data compendium 2008 edition. Table 2.1. Characteristics of nursing home residents in the United States, 2007. Available at:http://www.cms.hhs.gov/ Certification andComplianc/Downloads/2008NursingHomeDataCompendium_508.pdf. Accessed on February 25, 2009.
[63] Medicare home health agency utilization by State, calendar year 2006. Baltimore, MD: Centers for Medicare & Medicaid Services; 2006. Available at: www.cms.hhs.gov/ MedicareFeeforSvcPartsAB/Downloads/HHAst06.pdf. Accessed July 2009.
[64] Centers for Medicare & Medicaid Services. Table 8.1 Number of hospices, number of persons, covered days of care, total charges, and program payments for hospice services used by Medicare beneficiaries: calendar years 1993-2006. Health Care Finance Rev Stat Supp 2007. Available at: www.cms.hhs.gov/Medicare medicaid statsupp/ Downloads/2007table8.1b.pdf
[65] National health expenditures aggregate amounts and average percent change, by type of expenditure: selected calendar years 1960-2008. Baltimore, MD: Centers for Medicare & Medicaid Services; 2008. Available at: http://www.cms.hhs.gov/National Health ExpendData/ downloads/tables.pdf. Accessed on February 25, 2009.
[66] Medicare hospice data trends: 1998 - 2008. Baltimore, MD: Centers for Medicare & Medicaid Services; 2009. Available at: www.cms.hhs.gov/Hospice/downloads/Hospice _Data_1998-2008.zip.http://www.cms.hhs.gov/Hospice/downloads/Hospice_Data_ 1998-2008.zip. Accessed on December 2, 2009.
[67] Assistant Secretary for Planning and Evaluation, Office of Disability, Aging, and Long-Term Care Policy. Advance directives and advance care planning: report to Congress. Washington, DC: U.S. Department of Health and Human Services; 2008. Available at: http://aspe.hhs.gov/daltcp/reports/2008/adcongrpt.htm. Accessed on December 9, 2009.
[68] Field, M; Cassell, C. eds. *Approaching death: improving care at the end of life*. Washington, DC: National Academy Press; 1997.
[69] Connor, SR; Teno, J; Spence, C. et al. Family Evaluation of Hospice Care: results from voluntary submission of data via website. *J Pain Symptom Manage*, 2005 Jul, 30(1), 9-17.

3. PATIENT SAFETY

The Institute of Medicine (IOM) defines patient safety as "freedom from accidental injury due to medical care or medical errors."[1] In 1999, the IOM published *To Err Is Human: Building a Safer Health System*, which called for a national effort to reduce medical errors and improve patient safety.[1] Central to this effort is the ability to measure and track adverse events.

Measuring patient safety is complicated by difficulties in assessing and ensuring the systematic reporting medical errors and adverse events. All too often, adverse event reporting systems are laborious and cumbersome. Health care providers may also fear that if they participate in the analysis of medical errors or patient care processes, the findings may be used against them in court or harm their professional reputations Many factors limit the ability to aggregate data in sufficient numbers to rapidly identify prevalent risks and hazards in the delivery of patient care, their underlying causes, and practices that are most effective in mitigating them. These include difficulties aggregating and sharing data confidentially across facilities or State lines.

Despite these limitations, a better picture of patient safety is emerging. Progress has been made in recent years in raising awareness, developing reporting systems, and establishing national data collection standards. Examining patient safety using a combination of administrative data, medical record abstraction, spontaneous adverse event reports, and patient surveys allows a more robust understanding of what is improving and what is not. Still, data remain incomplete for a comprehensive national assessment of patient safety.[2]

Importance

Mortality

Number of Americans who die each year from
medical errors (1999 est.) .... 44,000-98,000[1]

Cost

Cost attributable to medical errors (lost income, disability,
and health care costs) (1999 est.)....................... ....$17 billion-$29 billion[1]
Annual cost attributable to surgical errors (2008 est.).............$1.5 billion[3]

Measures

This year's patient safety chapter highlights four core measures and seven additional measures related to health care-associated infections (HAIs), surgical complications, other complications of hospital care, and complications of medications:

Core measures are:

- Appropriate timing of antibiotics among surgical patients.
- Postoperative care composite: pneumonia or venous thromboembolic event.
- Adverse events associated with central venous catheters (CVCs).
- Potentially inappropriate prescription medications for adults age 65 and over.

Additional noncore measures include:

- Catheter-associated urinary tract infections (UTIs).

- Postoperative sepsis.
- Postoperative respiratory failure.
- Accidental puncture or laceration.
- Deaths following complications of care.
- Adverse drug events in the hospital.
- Patient safety culture composite.

Findings

Health Care-Associated Infections

Infections acquired during hospital care (nosocomial infections) are one of the most serious patient safety concerns. They are the most common complication of hospital care.[4] An estimated 1.7 million HAIs occur each year in hospitals, leading to about 100,000 deaths. The most common infections are urinary tract, surgical site, and bloodstream infections.[5]

A specific medical error cannot be identified in most cases of HAIs. However, better application of evidence-based preventive measures can reduce rates of HAIs within an institution. Such measures include using urinary catheters only when absolutely needed and administering prophylactic antibiotics before surgery at the right time.

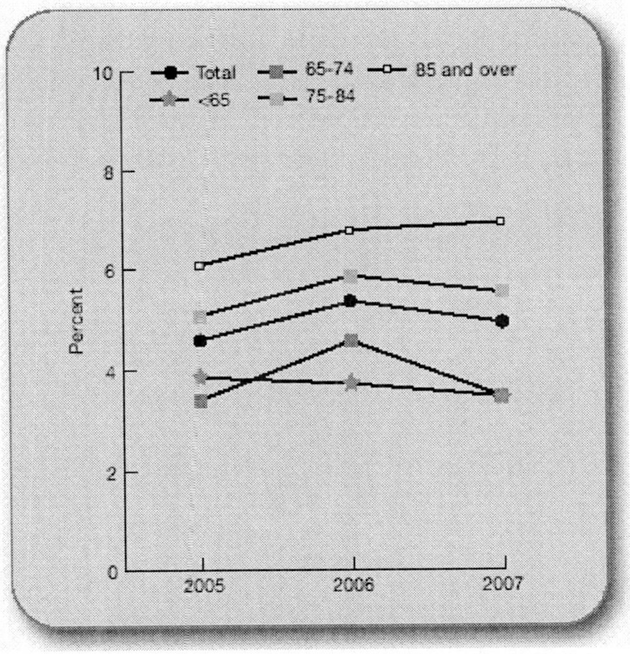

Source: Centers for Medicare & Medicaid Services, Medicare Patient Safety Monitoring System (MPSMS), 2005-2007.

Denominator: Adult hospitalized Medicare fee-for-service discharges from the MPSMS sample having major surgery and meeting specific criteria for each measure.

Figure 3.1. Adult Medicare surgery patients with postoperative catheter-associated urinary tract infection, overall and by age, 2005-2007

Outcome: Catheter-Associated Urinary Tract Infections

The urinary tract is a common site of HAI. Urinary catheter use and specific comorbid conditions can increase the risk of developing a UTI. Approximately 40% of all HAIs are attributed to catheter-associated UTIs.[6]

- In 2007, the total percentage of adult Medicare surgical patients with catheter-associated UTIs was 4.9% (Figure 3.1).
- From 2005 to 2007, there were no statistically significant changes overall or for any age group.
- In all 3 data years, surgery patients age 85 and over were more likely to have catheter-associated UTIs compared with patients under age 65.
- In 2006 and 2007, patients ages 75-84 were also more likely to have these infections compared with patients under age 65.

Prevention: Appropriate Timing of Antibiotics among Surgical Patients

Wound infection following surgery is a common HAI. Hospitals can reduce the risk of surgical site infection by making sure patients get the right antibiotics at the right time on the day of their surgery. Surgery patients who get antibiotics within the hour before their operation are less likely to get wound infections than those who do not. Getting an antibiotic earlier or after surgery begins is not as effective. However, taking these antibiotics for more than 24 hours after routine surgery is usually not necessary and can increase the risk of side effects, such as antibiotic resistance and serious types of diarrhea. Among adult Medicare patients having surgery, the National Healthcare Quality Report (NHQR) tracks receipt of antibiotics within 1 hour prior to surgical incision, discontinuation of antibiotics within 24 hours after end of surgery, and a composite of these two measures.

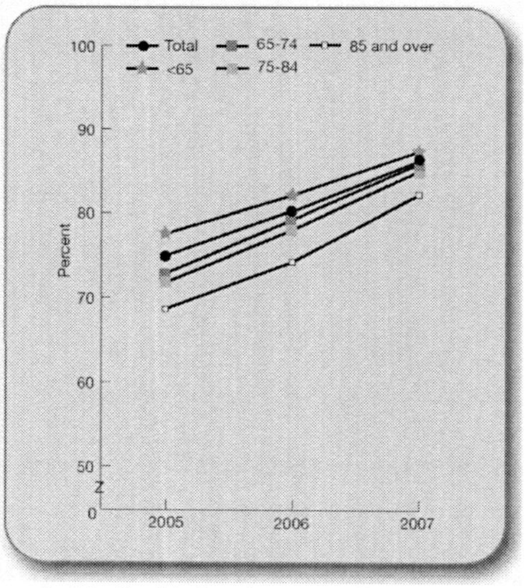

Source: Centers for Medicare & Medicaid Services, Medicare Quality Improvement Organization Program, 2005-2007.

Denominator: Hospitalized patients having surgery.

Figure 3.2. Adult surgery patients who received appropriate timing of antibiotics: Overall composite, by age, 2005-2007

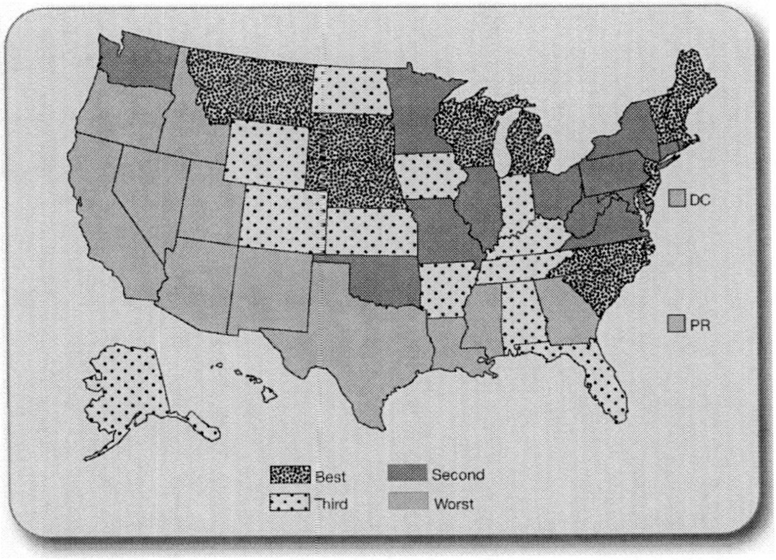

Key: Best quartile indicates States with highest rates of adult surgery patients who received appropriate timing of antibiotics; worst quartile indicates States with lowest rates.

Source: Centers for Medicare & Medicaid Services, Medicare Quality Improvement Organization Program, 2007.

Denominator: Hospitalized patients having surgery.

Figure 3.3. State variation: Adult surgery patients who received appropriate timing of antibiotics, 2007

- The percentage of adult surgery patients who received appropriate timing of antibiotics improved from 2005 (74.9%) to 2007 (86.4%) (Figure 3.2). Improvement was also seen among all age groups during this period.
- In all years, patients ages 65-74, 75-84, and 85 and over were less likely than patients under age 65 to receive appropriately timed antibiotics.
- The 13 States[XLVII] in the best quartile (highest rates of adult patients who received appropriate timing of antibiotics) in 2007 (Figure 3.3) had a combined average rate of 91.2%. These States are primarily located in New England and the Midwest.
- Eleven States,[XLVIII] the District of Columbia, and Puerto Rico were in the worst quartile (lowest rates) in 2007 and had a combined average rate of 80.5%. These States are primarily located in the West and Southwest.

Outcome: Postoperative Sepsis

Sepsis, a severe bloodstream infection, can occur after surgery. Rates can be reduced by giving patients appropriate prophylactic antibiotics 1 hour prior to surgical incision.

- From 2004 to 2006, the rate of postoperative sepsis increased from 13.2 to 15.1 per 1,000 elective surgery discharges of adults age 18 and over (Figure 3.4). Rates increased for patients with private insurance, Medicare, and Medicaid.
- In all years, patients with Medicare and Medicaid had higher rates of postoperative sepsis than patients with private insurance.

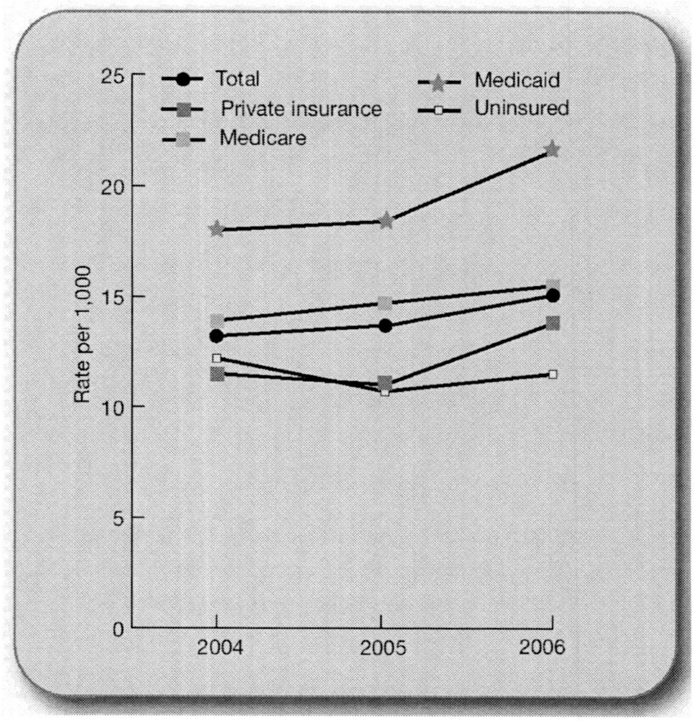

Source: Agency for Healthcare Research and Quality, Healthcare Cost and Utilization Project, Nationwide Inpatient Sample, 2004-2006.

Note: Rates are adjusted by age, gender, age-gender interactions, comorbidities, and diagnosis-related group clusters.

Figure 3.4. Postoperative sepsis after an operating room procedure per 1,000 elective surgery discharges, adults age 18 and over, 2004-2006

Surgical Care

Adverse health events can occur during episodes of care, especially during and soon after surgery. Although some events may be related to a patient's underlying condition, many can be avoided if appropriate care is provided.

Outcome: Postoperative Care Composite

Complications after surgery may include, but are not limited to, pneumonia and blood clots.

- From 2002 to 2007, the overall percentage of adult surgery patients who had postoperative pneumonia or a thromboembolic event decreased from 3.4% to 1.4%. During the same period, the percentage of adult surgery patients ages 65-74 and 75-84 with postoperative complications also decreased significantly (Figure 3.5).
- In all data years, adult surgery patients ages 75-84 were more likely to have postoperative complications compared with those ages 65-74.

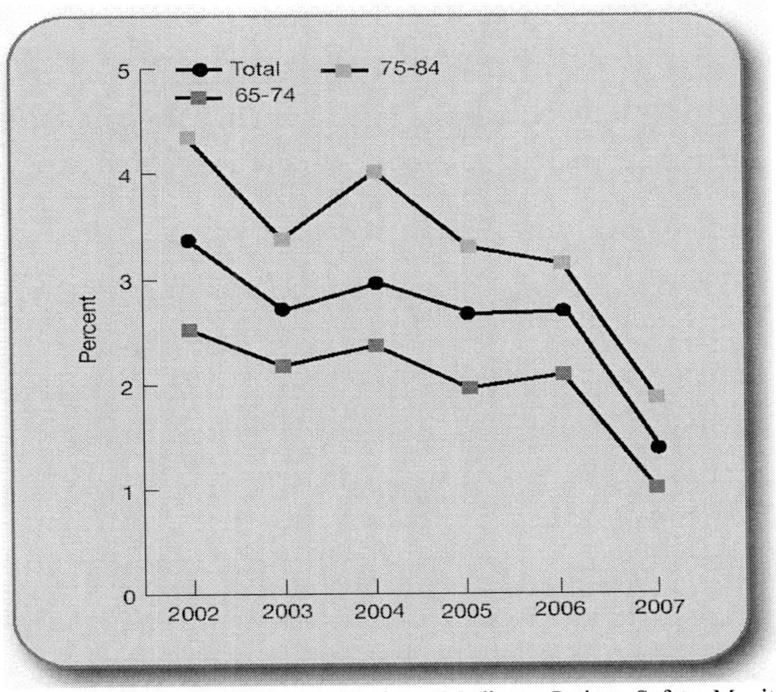

Source: Centers for Medicare & Medicaid Services, Medicare Patient Safety Monitoring System (MPSMS), 2002-2007.

Several measures related to heart disease are also presented in other chapters of this report. Timeliness of cardiac reperfusion for heart attack patients is tracked in Chapter 4, Timeliness, and receipt of complete written discharge instructions by patients with heart failure is tracked in Chapter 5, Patient Centeredness.

Adult hospitalized Medicare fee-for-service discharges from the MPSMS sample having major surgery and meeting specific criteria for each measure.

Figure 3.5. Composite measure: Adult Medicare surgery patients with postoperative complications (postoperative pneumonia or venous thromboembolic event), 2002-2007

Outcome: Postoperative Respiratory Failure

Respiratory failure is not uncommon after surgery and may necessitate reintubation or prolonged mechanical ventilation. Causes include oversedation, exacerbation of underlying cardiovascular or respiratory conditions, and ventilator-associated pneumonia. Although some cases of respiratory failure cannot be prevented, closer attention to risk factors can reduce rates within an institution.

- From 2004 to 2006, there were no statistically significant changes in rates of postoperative respiratory failure per 1,000 elective surgery discharges of adults age 18 and over for most insurance groups (Figure 3.6). However, for uninsured/self-pay patients, rates increased from 10.3 to 11.6.
- In all years, patients with Medicare and Medicaid had higher rates of postoperative respiratory failure than did patients with private insurance. In 2005 and 2006, rates were also higher among uninsured/self-pay patients than among patients with private insurance.

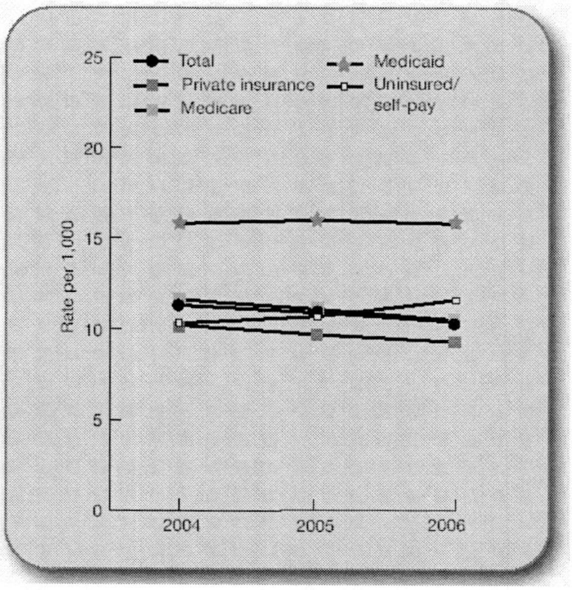

Source: Agency for Healthcare Research and Quality, Healthcare Cost and Utilization Project, Nationwide Inpatient Sample, 2004-2006.

Note: Rates are adjusted by age, gender, age-gender interactions, comorbidities, and diagnosis-related group clusters.

Figure 3.6. Postoperative respiratory failure per 1,000 elective surgery discharges after an operating room procedure, adults age 18 and over, 2004-2006

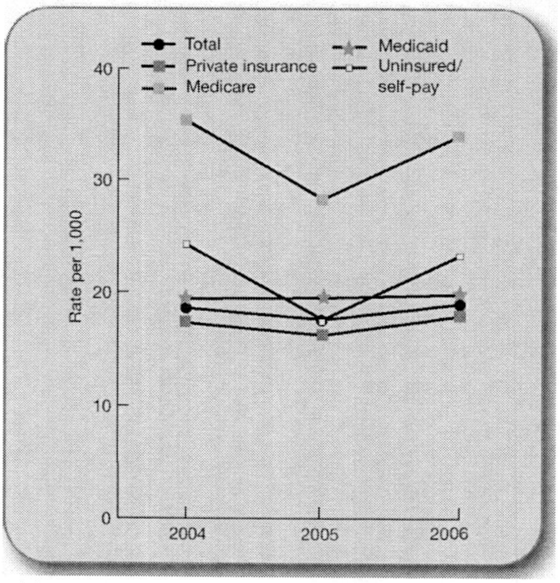

Source: Agency for Healthcare Research and Quality, Healthcare Cost and Utilization Project, Nationwide Inpatient Sample, 2004-2006.

Note: Rates are adjusted by age, gender, age-gender interactions, comorbidities, and diagnosis-related group clusters.

Figure 3.7. Postoperative respiratory failure per 1,000 elective surgery discharges after an operating room procedure, children under age 18, 2004-2006

- From 2004 to 2006, there were no statistically significant changes in rates of postoperative respiratory failure per 1,000 elective surgery discharges of children under age 18 overall or for any insurance group (Figure 3.7).
- In all years, pediatric patients with Medicare and Medicaid had higher rates of postoperative respiratory failure than patients with private insurance. Rates were also significantly higher among uninsured/self-pay patients in 2004 and 2006 than among those with private insurance.

Other Complications of Hospital Care

Besides surgery, other types of care delivered in hospitals can place patients at risk for injury or death.

Outcome: Adverse Events Associated with Central Venous Catheters

Patients who require a CVC to be inserted into or from the great vessels leading to the heart tend to be severely ill. However, the placement and use of these catheters can result in infections and other complications.

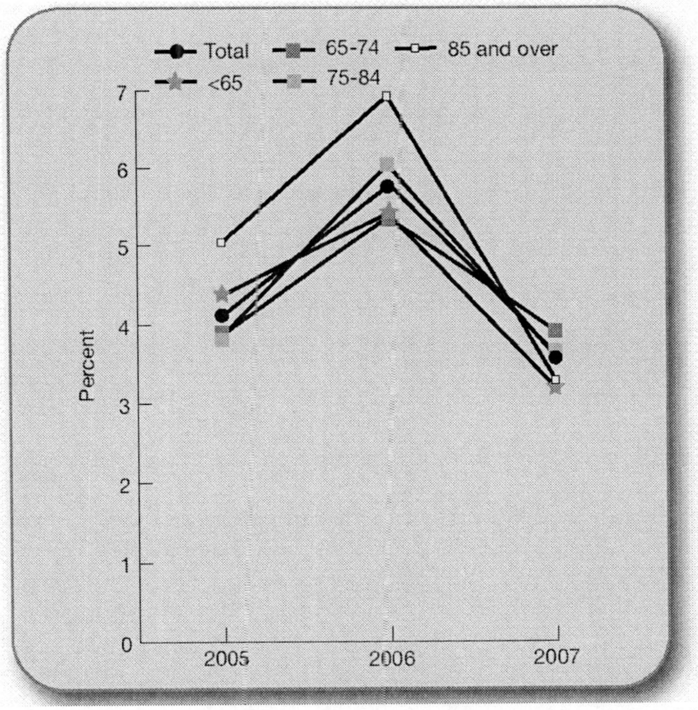

Source: Centers for Medicare & Medicaid Services, Medicare Patient Safety Monitoring System (MPSMS), 2005-2007.

Denominator: Adult hospitalized Medicare fee-for-service discharges from the MPSMS sample with CVC placement.

Note: Mechanical adverse events include allergic reaction (to the catheter), tamponade, perforation, pneumothorax, hematoma, shearing off of the catheter, air embolism, misplaced catheter, thrombosis or embolism, knotting of the pulmonary artery catheter, and certain other events.

Figure 3.8. Bloodstream infections or mechanical adverse events associated with central venous catheter placement: Overall composite, by age, 2005-2007

- From 2005 to 2007, there were no statistically significant changes overall or for any age group in the percentage of CVC placements with associated complications (Figure 3.8).

Outcome: Accidental Puncture or Laceration

Adverse events, including the nicking or cutting of bodily organs and blood vessels, are possible during any operation or procedure. This may be especially true in emergent situations, when, according to an expert panel review, some of these occurrences are not preventable. Puncture or laceration can lead to serious complications.[7]

- From 2004 to 2006, there were no statistically significant changes in the rate of accidental puncture or laceration during procedure for adults age 18 and over overall or for any insurance group (Figure 3.9).
- In all data years, those who were uninsured/self-pay/no charge were less likely to have accidental puncture or laceration during a procedure compared with all other insurance groups.

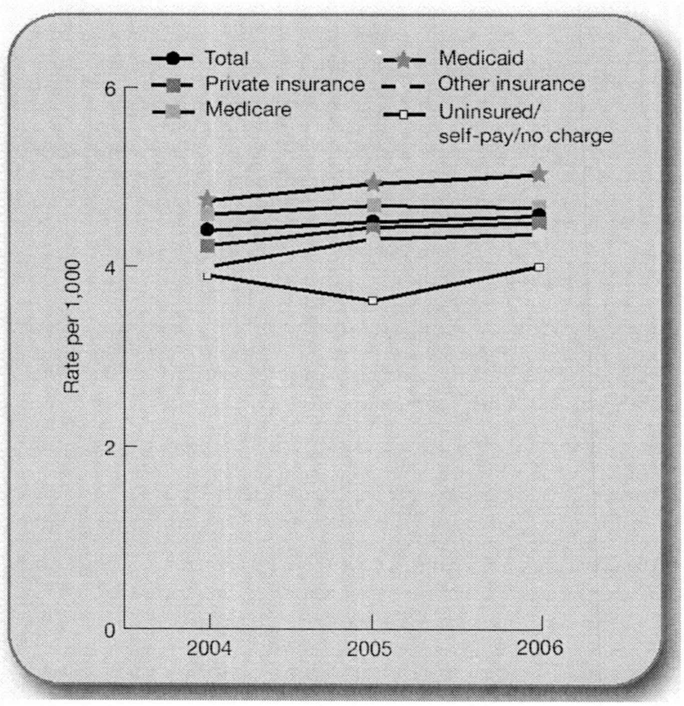

Source: Agency for Healthcare Research and Quality, Healthcare Cost and Utilization Project, Nationwide Inpatient Sample, 2004-2006.

Note: Rates are adjusted by age, gender, age-gender interactions, comorbidities, and diagnosis-related group clusters.

Figure 3.9. Accidental puncture or laceration during procedure per 1,000 discharges, adults age 18 over, 2004-2006

Outcome: Deaths Following Complications of Care

Many complications that arise during hospital stays cannot be prevented. However, rapid identification and aggressive treatment of complications may prevent these complications from leading to death. Deaths following complications of care, also called "failure to rescue," is an indicator that tracks deaths among patients whose hospitalizations are complicated by pneumonia, thromboembolic events, sepsis, acute renal failure, gastrointestinal bleeding or acute ulcer, shock, or cardiac arrest.[7]

- From 2004 to 2006, the rate of deaths following complications of care declined from 128.9 to 114.0 per 1,000 admissions of adults ages 18-74 (Figure 3.10). A significant decrease was also seen among all insurance groups during the same period.
- In all data years, uninsured individuals were more likely to have deaths potentially resulting from care compared with all other insurance groups.

Complications of Medications

Complications of medications are common safety problems. Some, but not all, adverse drug events may be related to misuse of medication. However, prescribing medications that are inappropriate for a specific population may increase the risk of adverse drug events.

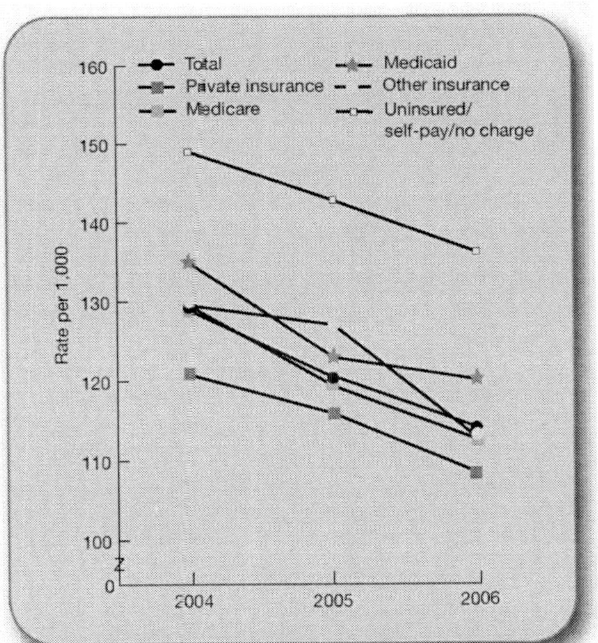

Source: Agency for Healthcare Research and Quality, Healthcare Cost and Utilization Project, Nationwide Inpatient Sample, 2004-2006.

Denominator: Patients ages 18-74 years from U.S. community hospitals whose hospitalizations are complicated by pneumonia, thromboembolic events, sepsis, acute renal failure, gastrointestinal bleeding or acute ulcer, shock, or cardiac arrest.

Note: Rates are adjusted by age, gender, comorbidities, and diagnosis-related group clusters.

Figure 3.10. Deaths per 1,000 discharges with complications potentially resulting from care (failure to rescue), adults ages 18-74, by insurance, 2004-2006

Outcome: Adverse Drug Events in the Hospital

Some medications used in hospitals can cause serious complications. The Medicare Patient Safety Monitoring System tracks a number of adverse drug events, including serious bleeding associated with intravenous heparin, low-molecular-weight heparin, or warfarin, and hypoglycemia associated with insulin or oral hypoglycemics.

- In 2007, adverse drug events in the hospital related to some frequently used medications ranged from 3.4% of Medicare patients who received low-molecular-weight heparin to 8.9% of Medicare patients who received intravenous heparin (Figure 3.11).
- The rates of each adverse drug event decreased significantly from 2004 to 2007.

Outcome: Potentially Inappropriate Prescription Medications for Adults Age 65 and Over

Some drugs are considered potentially harmful for older patients but nevertheless were prescribed to them.[8],[XLIX]

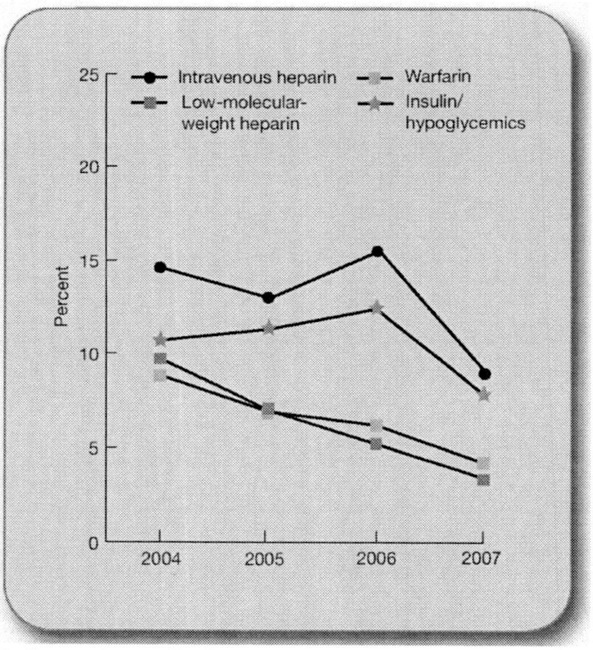

Source: Centers for Medicare & Medicaid Services, Medicare Patient Safety Monitoring System (MPSMS), 2004-2007.

Denominator: Adult hospitalized Medicare fee-for-service discharges from the MPSMS sample receiving specified medication.

Figure 3.11. Hospitalized Medicare patients with adverse drug events, 2004-2007

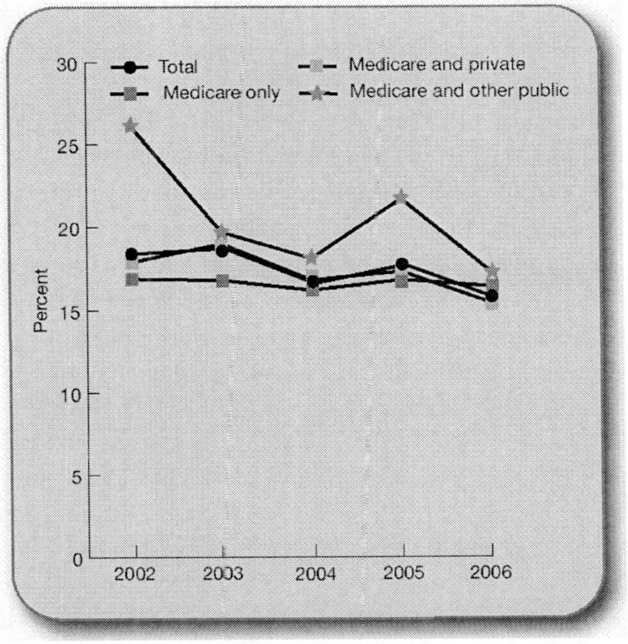

Source: Agency for Healthcare Research and Quality, Medical Expenditure Panel Survey, 2002-2006.
Denominator: Civilian noninstitutionalized population age 65 and over.
Note: Prescription medications received include all prescribed medications initially purchased or otherwise obtained, as well as any refills.

Figure 3.12. Adults age 65 and over who received potentially inappropriate prescription medications in the calendar year, 2002-2006

- From 2002 to 2006, the percentage of older patients who reported purchasing at least 1 of 33 potentially inappropriate drugs decreased significantly, from 18.4% to 15.7% (Figure 3.12).
- From 2002 to 2006, the rate of patients who received potentially inappropriate medication decreased significantly among those with Medicare and private insurance or Medicare and other public insurance.

Focus on Patient Safety Culture

High-reliability organizations that achieve low rates of adverse events establish "cultures of safety." A culture of safety is characterized by shared dedication to making work safe, blame-free reporting and communication about error, collaboration and teamwork across disciplines, and adequate resources to prevent adverse events. AHRQ developed the Hospital Survey on Patient Safety Culture to help hospitals assess the culture of safety in their facilities. AHRQ began producing comparative database reports in 2007 to help hospitals assess their performance relative to similar institutions.

In this NHQR, we present data from the Hospital Survey on Patient Safety Culture: 2009 Comparative Database Report.[9] This chapter is based on survey responses collected in 2008 from nearly 200,000 hospital staff in 622 hospitals. The average hospital response rate was 52%, with an average of 316 completed surveys per hospital. Most hospitals administered paper surveys rather than Web-based surveys. In addition, most hospitals administered the survey to all staff or a sample of all staff from all hospital departments.

Nurses accounted for more than one-third of respondents, followed by "other." More than three-quarters of respondents had direct interaction with patients.

Results are presented for the 12 patient safety culture composites addressed in the survey, expressed as average percent positive response. Percent positive refers to the percentage of responses that agree or strongly agree with a positively worded item (e.g., "People support one another in this work area") and the percentage that disagree or disagree strongly with a negatively worded item (e.g., "We have safety problems in this work area"). Hospitals contributing data to the comparative database mirror the population of U.S. hospitals as a whole, but participation is entirely voluntary. Thus, findings may not be generalizable to all types of facilities.

- A strength for most hospitals was Teamwork Within Units, the extent to which staff support each other, treat each other with respect, and work together as a team.
- Many hospitals performed poorly on Nonpunitive Response to Error, the extent to which staff feel that their mistakes and event reports are not held against them and that mistakes are not kept in their personnel file. Similar results were seen for Handoffs and Transitions, the extent to which important patient care information is transferred across hospital units and during shift changes.

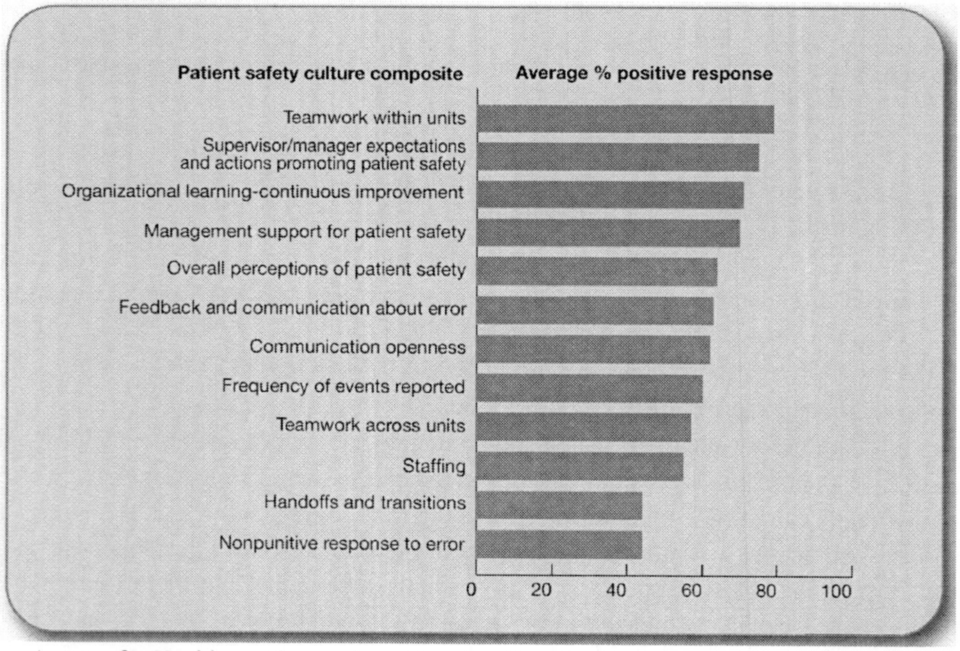

Source: Agency for Healthcare Research and Quality, Hospital Survey on Patient Safety Culture: 2009 Comparative DatabaseReport.

Figure 3.13. Patient safety culture composites, all hospitals, 2008

References

[1] Kohn, L; Corrigan, J; Donaldson, M. eds. *To err is human: building a safer health system*. Washington, DC: Institute of Medicine, Committee on Quality of Health Care in America; 2000.

[2] Aspden, P; Corrigan, J; Wolcott, J. et al. *Patient safety: achieving a new standard of care*. Washington, DC: Institute of Medicine, Committee on Data Standards for Patient Safety; 2004.

[3] Encinosa, WE; Hellinger, FJ. The impact of medical errors on ninety-day costs and outcomes: an examination of surgical patients. *Health Serv Res,* 2008 Dec, 43(6), 2067-85. Epub 2008 Jul 25.

[4] Thomas, EJ; Studdert, DM; HR, B. et al. Incidence and types of adverse events and negligent care in Utah and Colorado. *Med Care,* 2000, 38, 261-71.

[5] Klevens, RM; Edwards, JR; Richards, CL. et al. Estimating health care-associated infections and deaths in U.S. hospitals, 2002. *Pub Hlth Rep,* 2007, 122, 160-5.

[6] Tambyah, PA; Maki, DG. Catheter-associated urinary tract infection is rarely symptomatic: a prospective study of 1,497 catheterized patients. *Arch Intern Med,* 2000 Mar 13, 160(5), 678-82.

[7] Guide to Patient Safety Indicators Version 3.1. Rockville, MD: Agency for Healthcare Research and Quality; 2003. Available at: http://www.qualityindicators.ahrq.gov/downloads/psi/word/psi_guide_v31.doc. Accessed on November 17, 2009.

[8] Zhan, C; Sangl, J; Bierman, AS. et al. Potentially inappropriate medication use in the community-dwelling elderly: findings from the 1996 Medical Expenditure Panel Survey. *JAMA,* 2001 Dec 12, 286(22), 2823-9.

[9] Hospital Survey on Patient Safety Culture. 2009 comparative database report. Rockville, MD: Agency for Healthcare Research and Quality; 2009. AHRQ Publication No. 09-0030. Available at: http://www.ahrq.gov/qual/hospsurvey09/. Accessed on June 15, 2009.

4. Timeliness

Timeliness is the health care system's capacity to provide health care quickly after a need is recognized. It is one of the six dimensions of quality the Institute of Medicine established as a priority for improvement in the health care system.[1] Measures of timeliness include time spent waiting in doctors' offices and emergency departments (EDs) and the interval between identifying a need for specific tests and treatments and actually receiving those services.

Importance

Morbidity and Mortality

- Lack of timeliness can result in emotional distress, physical harm, and higher treatment costs for patients.[2,3]

- Stroke patients' mortality and long-term disability are largely influenced by the timeliness of therapy.[4,5]
- Timely delivery of appropriate care can help reduce mortality and morbidity for chronic conditions, such as kidney disease.[6]
- Timeliness in childhood immunizations helps maximize the protection from vaccine-preventable diseases while minimizing risks to the child and reducing the chance of disease outbreaks.[7]
- Timely antibiotic treatments are associated with improved clinical outcomes.[8]

Cost

- Early care for comorbid conditions has been shown to reduce hospitalization rates and costs for Medicare beneficiaries.[9]
- Some research suggests that, over the course of 30 years, the costs of treating diabetic complications can approach $50,000 per patient.[10] Early care for complications in patients with diabetes can reduce overall costs of the disease.[11]
- Timely outpatient care can reduce admissions for pediatric asthma, which in 2003 accounted for more than $1.25 billion in hospitalization charges.[12,13]

Measures

This chapter focuses on two core report measures related to timeliness of primary, emergency, and hospital care:

- Getting care for illness or injury as soon as wanted.
- ED visits in which patients left without being seen.

In addition, one noncore measure is presented:

- Timeliness of cardiac reperfusion for heart attack patients.

Findings

Getting Care for Illness or Injury as Soon as Wanted

A patient's primary care provider should be the first point of contact for most illnesses and injuries. A patient's ability to receive timely treatment for illness and injury is a key element in a patient-centered health care system.

- From 2002 to 2006, there were no statistically significant changes in the percentages of adults ages 18 to 64 and age 65 and over who needed care right away for an illness, injury, or condition in the last 12 months who sometimes or never got care as soon as wanted (Figure 4.1). This was also true for all insurance groups.

- In all years, the percentage of adults ages 18-64 who sometimes or never got care as soon as wanted was higher for those with public insurance or no insurance than for those with private insurance.
- In 2006, among children who needed care right away for an illness, injury, or condition in the last 12 months, 7.1% sometimes or never got care as soon as wanted (Figure 4.2). Between 2002 and 2006, there were no statistically significant changes in this percentage overall or for any insurance group.
- In all data years, children who had public insurance were more likely to sometimes or never get care as soon as wanted than those with private insurance.

Emergency Department Visits in Which Patients Left without Being Seen

In 2006, an estimated 119.2 million visits were made to hospital EDs compared with 110.2 million visits in 2004.[14,15] The median waiting time for patients to be seen by a physician during an ED visit in the United States was 31 minutes.[14]

Not all patients seeking care in an ED need urgent care, and use of EDs for nonurgent care leads to longer waiting times. Although many factors may lead a patient seeking care in a hospital ED to leave without being seen, long waits tend to exacerbate the problem. Note that our measure of leaving an ED without being seen does not distinguish between appropriate and inappropriate use of the ED.

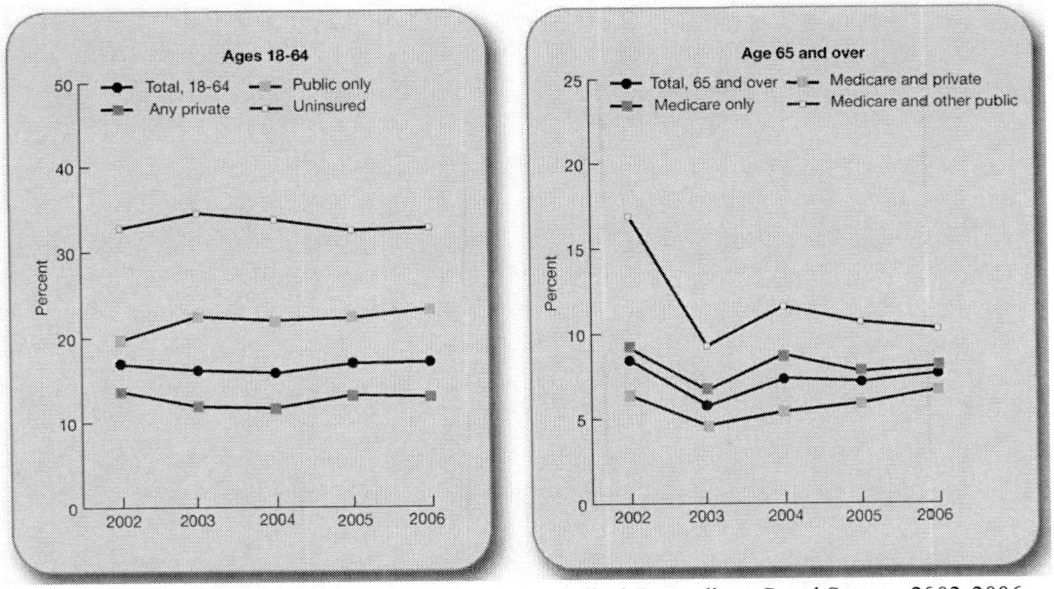

Source: Agency for Healthcare Research and Quality, Medical Expenditure Panel Survey, 2002-2006. Denominator: Civilian noninstitutionalized population age 18 and over.

Figure 4.1. Adults who needed care right away for an illness, injury, or condition in the last 12 months who s ometimes or never got care as soon as wanted, by insurance, 2002-2006

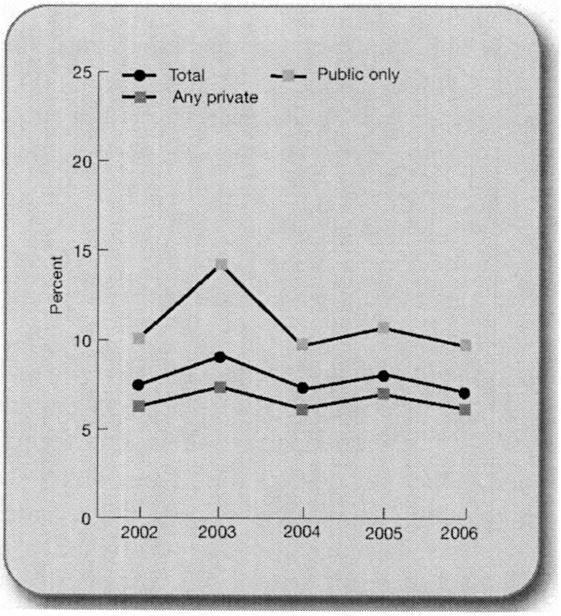

Source: Agency for Healthcare Research and Quality, Medical Expenditure Panel Survey, 2002-2006.
Denominator: Civilian noninstitutionalized population under age 18.

Figure 4.2. Children who needed care right away for an illness, injury, or condition in the last 12 months who sometimes or never got care as soon as wanted, by insurance, 2002-2006

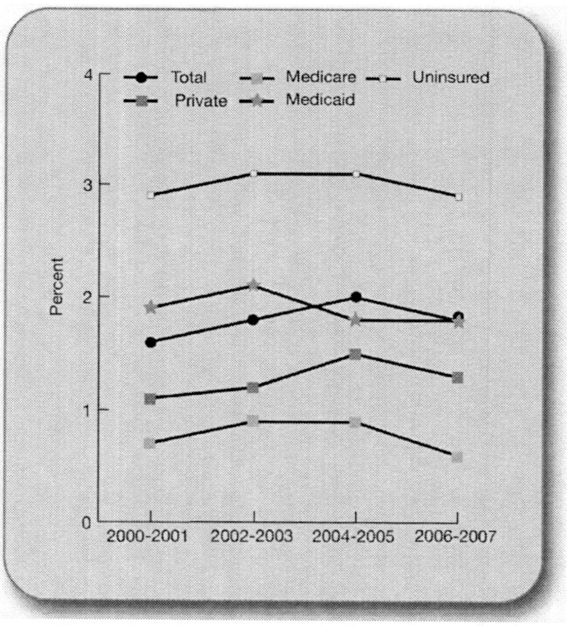

Source: Centers for Disease Control and Prevention, National Center for Health Statistics, National Hospital Ambulatory Medical Care Survey, 2000-2007.
Denominator: Visits to EDs of general and short-stay hospitals.

Figure 4.3. Emergency department visits in which patients left without being seen, by insurance, 2000-2007

- From 2000-2001 to 2006-2007, the percentage of ED visits in which patients left without being seen did not change significantly overall or for any insurance group (Figure 4.3).
- In all years, patients with Medicaid and patients with no health insurance were more likely to leave without being seen than patients with private health insurance.

Timeliness of Cardiac Reperfusion for Heart Attack Patients

The capacity to treat hospital patients in a timely fashion is especially important for emergency situations, such as heart attacks. Some heart attacks are caused by blood clots. Early actions, such as percutaneous coronary intervention (PCI) or fibrinolytic medication, may open blockages caused by blood clots, reduce heart muscle damage, and save lives.[16] To be effective, these actions need to be performed quickly after the start of a heart attack.

In this chapter, we introduce two new measures of timeliness of cardiac reperfusion:

- PCI within 90 minutes among appropriate patients.
- Fibrinolytic medication within 30 minutes among appropriate patients.
- Among heart attack patients, the percentage of patients receiving PCI within 90 minutes improved from 42.1% in 2005 to 71.8% in 2007 (Figure 4.4).
- The percentage of patients receiving fibrinolytic medication within 30 minutes improved from 37.9% to 50.0%.

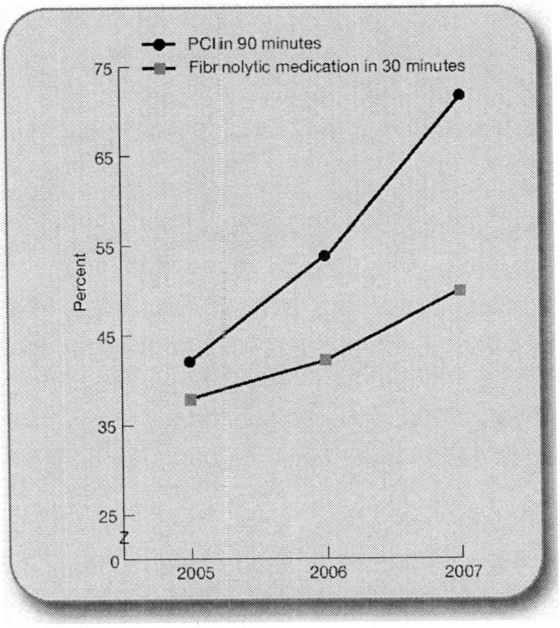

Key: PCI = percutaneous coronary intervention.

Source: Centers for Medicare & Medicaid Services, Medicare Quality Improvement Organization Program, 2005-2007.

Denominator: Patients hospitalized with a principal diagnosis of acute myocardial infarction who were appropriate candidates for PCI or fibrinolytic medication.

Figure 4.4. Hospital patients with heart attack who received PCI within 90 minutes or fibrinolytic medication within 30 minutes, 2005-2007

REFERENCES

[1] Institute of Medicine Committee on Quality of Health Care in America. Crossing the quality chasm: a new health system for the 21st century. Washington, DC: National Academies Press; 2001.

[2] Leddy, KM; Kaldenberg, DO; Becker, BW. Timeliness in ambulatory care treatment. An examination of patient satisfaction and wait times in medical practices and outpatient test and treatment facilities. *J Ambul Care Manage,* 2003 Apr-Jun, 26(2), 138-49.

[3] Boudreau, RM; McNally, C; Rensing, EM. et al. Improving the timeliness of written patient notification of mammography results by mammography centers. *Breast J,* 2004 Jan-Feb, 10(1), 10-19.

[4] Schellinger, PD; Warach, S. Therapeutic time window of thrombolytic therapy following stroke. *Curr Atheroscler Rep,* 2004 Jul, 6(4), 288-94.

[5] Kwan, J; Hand, P; Sandercock, P. Improving the efficiency of delivery of thrombolysis for acute stroke: a systematic review. *QJM,* 2004 May, 97(5), 273-9.

[6] Kinchen, KS; Sadler, J; Fink, N. et al. The timing of specialist evaluation in chronic kidney disease and mortality. *Ann Intern Med,* 2002 Sep 17, 137(6), 479-86.

[7] Luman, ET; Barker, LE; Shaw, KM. et al. Timeliness of childhood vaccinations in the United States: days undervaccinated and number of vaccines delayed. *JAMA,* 2005 Mar 9, 293(10), 1204-11.

[8] Houck, PM; Bratzler, DW. Administration of first hospital antibiotics for community-acquired pneumonia: does timeliness affect outcomes? *Curr Opin Infect Dis,* 2005 Apr, 18(2), 151-6.

[9] Himelhoch, S; Weller, WE; Wu, AW. et al. Chronic medical illness, depression, and use of acute medical services among Medicare beneficiaries. *Med Care,* 2004 Jun, 42(6), 512-21.

[10] Caro, JJ; Ward, AJ; O'Brien, JA. Lifetime costs of complications resulting from type 2 diabetes in the U.S. *Diabetes Care,* 2002 Mar, 25(3), 476-81.

[11] Ramsey, SD; Newton, K; Blough, D. et al. Patient-level estimates of the cost of complications in diabetes in a managed-care population. *Pharmacoeconomics,* 1999 Sep, 16(3), 285-95.

[12] Mellon, M; Parasuraman, B. Pediatric asthma: improving management to reduce cost of care. *J Manag Care Pharm,* 2004 Mar-Apr;10(2), 130-41.

[13] Calculated from Web site. Agency for Healthcare Research and Quality. Healthcare Cost and Utilization Project Kids' Inpatient Database. Available at: http://hcupnet.ahrq.gov/. Accessed on April 24, 2009.

[14] Pitts, S; Niska, R & Xu, J. et al. *National Hospital Ambulatory Medical Care Survey: 2006 emergency department summary*. National Health Statistics Reports, No. 7. Hyattsville, MD: National Center for Health Statistics; 2008. Available at: http://www.cdc.gov/nchs/data/nhsr/nhsr007.pdf. Accessed on July 7, 2009.

[15] McCaig, L. Nawar, E. *National Hospital Ambulatory Medical Care Survey: 2004 emergency department summary*. Advance Data From Vital and Health Statistics, No 372. Hyattsville, MD: National Center for Health Statistics; 2006. Available at: http://www.cdc.gov/nchs/data/ad/ad372.pdf. Accessed on November 5, 2008.

[16] Kloner, RA; Rezkalla, SH. Cardiac protection during acute myocardial infarction: where do we stand in 2004? *J Am Coll Cardiol*, 2004 Jul 21, 44(2), 276-86.

5. Patient Centeredness

Patient centeredness is defined as:

> [H]ealth care that establishes a partnership among practitioners, patients, and their families (when appropriate) to ensure that decisions respect patients' wants, needs, and preferences and that patients have the education and support they need to make decisions and participate in their own care.[1]

An important dimension of quality, patient centeredness "encompasses qualities of compassion, empathy, and responsiveness to the needs, values, and expressed preferences of the individual patient."[2] In addition, effective communication between the provider and the patient is often a legal requirement.[L]

Importance and Measures

Morbidity and Mortality

- Patient-centered approaches to care have been shown to improve patients' health status. These approaches rely on building a provider-patient relationship, improving communication, fostering a positive atmosphere, and encouraging patients to actively participate in provider-patient interactions.[3,4]
- A patient-centered approach has been shown to lessen patients' symptom burden.[5]
- Patient-centered care encourages patients to comply with treatment regimens.[6]
- Patient-centered care can reduce the chance of misdiagnosis due to poor communication.[7]

Cost

- Patient centeredness has been shown to reduce underuse and overuse of medical services.[8]
- Patient centeredness can reduce the strain on system resources and save money by reducing the number of diagnostic tests and referrals.[5]
- Although some studies have shown that being patient centered reduces medical costs and use of health service resources, others have shown that patient centeredness increases providers' costs, especially in the short run.[9]

Measures

The National Healthcare Quality Report (NHQR) tracks several measures of patients' experience of care. The core report measure is a composite of these measures—patients' assessments of how often their provider listened carefully to them, explained things clearly, respected what they had to say, and spent enough time with them. This measure is presented separately for adult and child patients. In addition, this NHQR includes a section focusing on care coordination.

Findings

Patients' Experience of Care—Adults

Optimal health care requires good communication between patients and providers, yet barriers to provider-patient communication are common. To provide all patients with the best possible care, providers must be able to understand patients' diverse health care needs and preferences and communicate clearly with patients about their care.

- From 2002 to 2006, the percentage of adults ages 18-64 with a doctor's office or clinic visit who reported poor communication decreased from 11.6% to 10.4% (Figure 5.1).

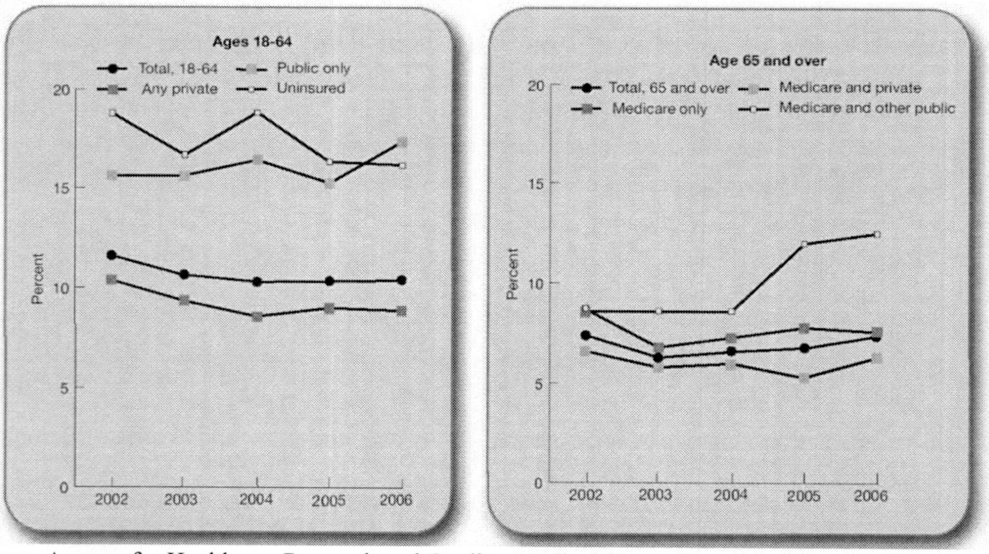

Source: Agency for Healthcare Research and Quality, Medical Expenditure Panel Survey, 2002-2006.

Denominator: Civilian noninstitutionalized population age 18 and over who had a doctor's office or clinic visit in the last 12 months.

Note: Patients who report that their health providers sometimes or never listened carefully, explained things clearly, showed respect for what they had to say, or spent enough time with them are considered to have poor communication.

Figure 5.1. Adults who had a doctor's office or clinic visit in the last 12 months who reported poor communication with health providers: Overall composite, by insurance, 2002-2006

- Between 2002 and 2006, the percentage of adults with a doctor's office or clinic visit who reported poor communication decreased for adults with any private insurance, from 10.4% to 8.9%.
- In all data years, adults with public insurance and uninsured adults were more likely to report poor communication with their health providers compared with those with private insurance.
- From 2002 to 2006, there were no statistically significant changes overall or for any insurance group in the percentage of adults age 65 and over with a doctor's office or clinic visit who reported poor communication with their health providers.
- In 2003, 2005, and 2006, adults with Medicare and other public insurance were more likely to report poor communication with their health providers compared with those with Medicare and private insurance.

Patients' Experience of Care—Children

Communication in children's health care can pose a particular challenge. Children are often less able to express their health care needs and preferences, and a third party (e.g., a parent or guardian) is involved in communication and decisionmaking. Optimal communication in children's health care can therefore have a significant impact on receipt of high-quality care and subsequent health status.

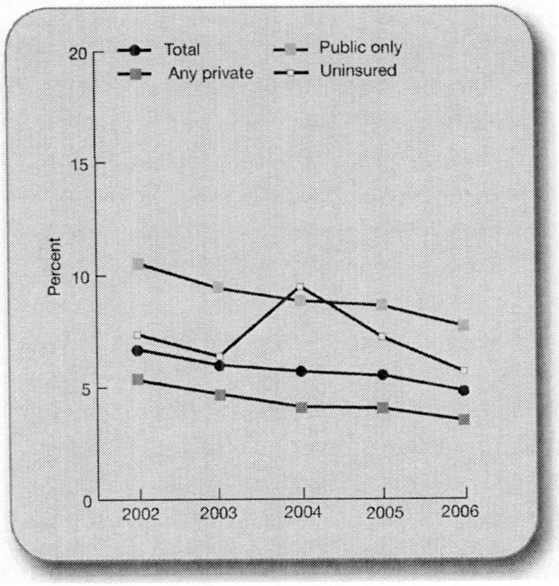

Source: Agency for Healthcare Research and Quality, Medical Expenditure Panel Survey, 2002-2006.

Denominator: Civilian noninstitutionalized population under age 18 who had a doctor's office or clinic visit in the last 12 months.

Note: Parents who report that their child's health providers sometimes or never listened carefully, explained things clearly, showed respect for what they had to say, or spent enough time with them are considered to have poor communication.

Figure 5.2. Children who had a doctor's office or clinic visit in the last 12 months whose parents reported poor communication with health providers: Overall composite, by insurance, 2002-2006

- In 2006, 4.8% of parents of children who had a doctor's office or clinic visit in the last 12 months reported poor communication with health providers. This rate is a significant improvement over the 2002 rate of 6.7% (Figure 5.2).
- Improvement since 2002 is also significant for children with any private insurance or public insurance only.
- In all data years, parents of children with public insurance were more likely to report poor communication with their health providers compared with those with private insurance.

Focus on Care Coordination

Health care in the United States was not designed to be patient centered. Clinical services are frequently organized around specific symptoms or organ systems and can be fragmented and difficult to navigate. Patients often receive medical services, treatments, and advice from multiple providers in many different care settings, each scrutinizing a particular body part and none attending to the patient as a whole. Communication of important information among providers and between providers and patients may entail delays or inaccuracies or fail to occur at all.

The patient-centered medical home is one approach to organizing care around a person and helping each person stay as healthy as possible. A key element is a personal physician leading a team of health care professionals. These professionals collectively take responsibility for providing all the services that a patient needs or arranging for and coordinating care provided by others.

This section focuses on the work of providers related to coordinating care. Care coordination is defined as the deliberate organization of patient care activities between two or more participants involved in a patient's care to facilitate appropriate delivery of health care services.[10] It is multidimensional and essential to preventing adverse events, ensuring efficiency, and making care patient centered.[10,11] Key elements of care coordination include integrating medical information from all the providers a patient sees and managing patient transitions from one setting of care to another.

The focus on care coordination in this NHQR does not attempt to provide a comprehensive framework for care coordination, nor does it provide an exhaustive list of potential measures. Rather, it provides examples where some information is available. AHRQ hopes that this section will stimulate productive discussions in the area of care coordination, including development and use of valid, reliable, and feasible quality measures. AHRQ intends this chapter to be the first step in an evolving national discussion on measuring care coordination.

Integration of Information

Patients often seek care from many providers. Medical information generated in different settings may not be sent to a patient's primary care provider. Actively gathering and managing all of a patient's medical information is an important part of care coordination. Tasks include ensuring that patients are informed of important findings such as test results, primary care doctors are informed of care from specialists, and providers within a practice have access to needed information.

No national survey currently gathers information from patients about these aspects of care coordination. To help fill this gap, we examined subnational data-gathering activities and identified the Massachusetts Health Quality Partners (MHQP) Patient Experience Survey as a unique source of this information. MHQP is an independent organization established in 1995. It is a broad-based coalition of physicians, hospitals, health plans, purchasers, consumers, academics, and government agencies working together to promote improvement in the quality of health care services in Massachusetts. MHQP has conducted the Patient Experience Survey since 2005.

In 2007, MHQP conducted a mail and Internet survey of commercially insured adult and pediatric patients' experiences of care. The survey included patients being served in primary care practices with at least three doctors.[12] Several questions related directly to coordination of information across providers and patients.

The survey was completed by 51,000 adult patients and 20,000 parents of pediatric patients receiving care in more than 400 medical practices in Massachusetts. The response rate was 42%.

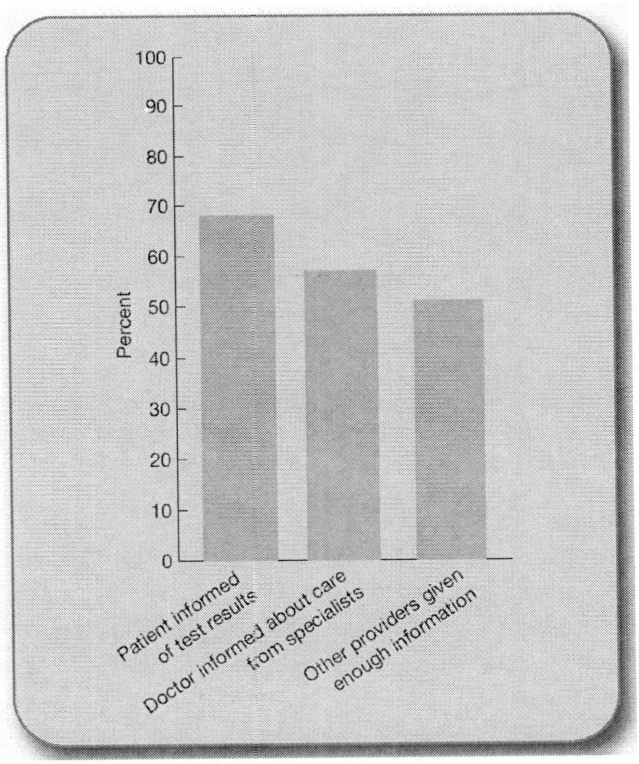

Source: Massachusetts Health Quality Partners, Patient Experience Survey, 2007.

Denominator: Commercially insured adults ages 18-64 in primary care practices with at least three doctors.

Note: Respondents limited to patients who received particular services in the past year: had a test, had a referral to a specialist, or saw another provider in their doctor's office.

Figure 5.3. Patients who reported that they always received test results, that their personal doctor always seemed informed and up to date about care received from specialist doctors, and that other providers at their doctor's office always had all the information they needed, commercially insured adults ages 18-64, Massachusetts, 2007

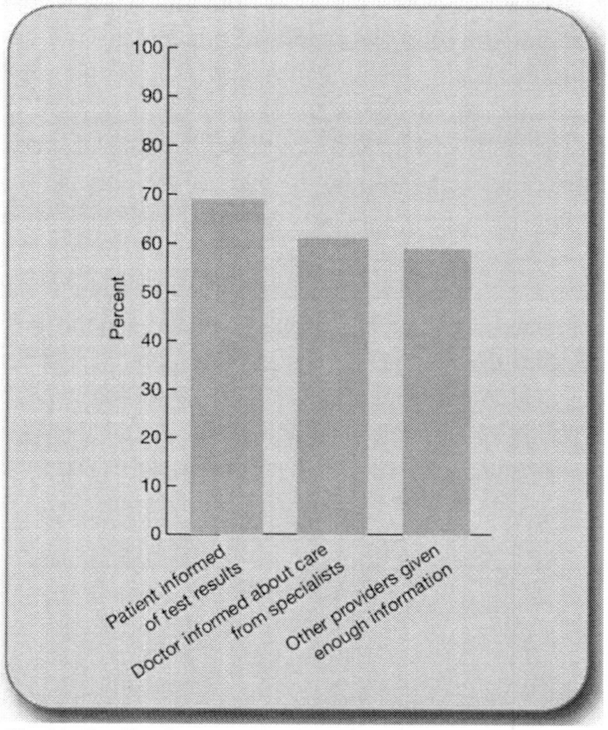

Source: Massachusetts Health Quality Partners, Patient Experience Survey, 2007.

Denominator: Commercially insured children under age 18 in primary care practices with at least three doctors.

Note: Respondents limited to parents of patients who received particular services in the past year: had a test, had a referral to a specialist, or saw another provider in their doctor's office.

Figure 5.4. Parents who reported that they always received test results for their child, that their child's personal doctor always seemed informed and up to date about care received from specialist doctors, and that other providers at their child's doctor's office always had all the information they needed, commercially insured children under age 18, Massachusetts, 2007

- Of adult patients who were sent for a blood test, x-ray, or other test by their personal primary care doctor, 68% reported that someone from the doctor's office always followed up to give them the test results (Figure 5.3).
- Of patients whose personal doctor recommended that they see a specialist, 57% reported that their doctor always seemed informed and up to date about the care they received from specialists.
- Among adults who saw other doctors or nurses in their personal doctor's office, 51% reported that the other providers always had all the information they needed to correctly diagnose and treat their health problem.
- Among parents of pediatric patients who were sent for a test, 69% reported that someone from the doctor's office always followed up to give the test results (Figure 5.4).
- Sixty-one percent of parents reported that their child's doctor always seemed informed and up to date about the care the child received from specialists.
- Among parents of pediatric patients who saw other doctors or nurses, 59% reported that the other providers always had all the information they needed.

Transitions of Care

As health care conditions and needs change, patients often need to be moved from one setting to another. These transitions of care place patients at heightened risk of adverse events. Important information may be lost or miscommunicated as responsibility is delivered to new parties.

A common transition of care is discharge from the hospital, with approximately 39 million community hospital discharges occurring each year.[13] Discharge from a hospital typically indicates improvement in a patient's condition so that the patient no longer requires inpatient care. It also means that the patient and family must resume responsibility for the patient's daily activities, diet, medications, and other treatments. The patient also needs to visit his or her personal doctor and know what to do if his or her condition deteriorates.

Discharge instructions can help ensure that a patient receives the information needed to stay healthy after leaving the hospital. The NHQR reports on a measure that tracks receipt of written discharge instructions among adult patients hospitalized for heart failure. It also reports on two measures that reflect discharged patients' perceptions regarding the adequacy of the discharge information they received.

- From 2005 to 2007, the percentage of hospitalized adult patients with heart failure who were given complete written discharge instructions improved from 57.5% to 76.0% (Figure 5.5). Improvements were observed among all age groups.
- Differences among age groups were not observed.

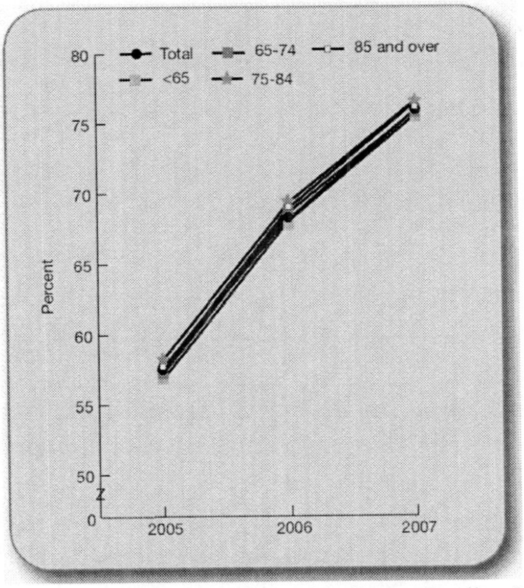

Source: Centers for Medicare & Medicaid Services, Medicare Quality Improvement Organization Program, 2005-2007.

Denominator: Hospitalized adult patients with a principal discharge diagnosis of heart failure.

Note: Complete written discharge instructions needed to address all of the following: activity level, diet, discharge medications, followup appointment, weight monitoring, and actions to take if symptoms worsen.

Figure 5.5. Hospitalized adult patients with heart failure who were given complete written discharge instructions, by age, 2005-2007

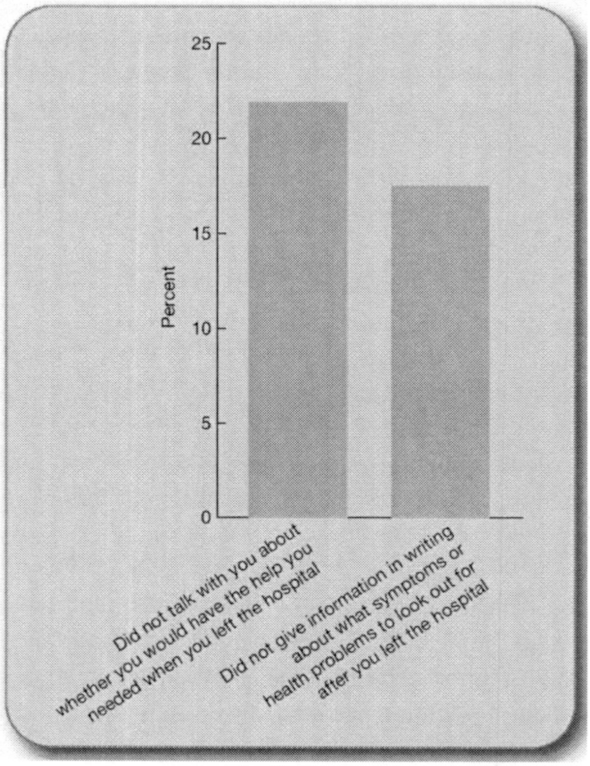

Source: Centers for Medicare & Medicaid Services, Medicare Quality Improvement Organization Program, 2008.

Denominator: Adult hospital patients.

Note: Rate is adjusted for patient mix, mode of data collection, and nonresponse bias.

Figure 5.6. Adult hospital patients who were discharged and reported that hospital staff did NOT provide adequate discharge information, 2008

- Among adult hospital patients, 21.9% reported that hospital staff did not talk with them about help at home and 17.5% reported that they did not get written information about what symptoms or problems to look for (Figure 5.6).

Care Coordination for Children with Special Health Care Needs

Children with special health care needs are those who have or are at increased risk for a chronic physical, developmental, behavioral, or emotional condition and who also require health and related services of a type or amount beyond that required by children generally.[14] They may need services not only from medical specialists, but also from other therapists (e.g., nutritionists, occupational therapists, mental health care providers) and educational specialists. Therefore, appropriate and timely coordination of care across multiple providers may be particularly important for children with special health care needs.

In the 2008 National Healthcare Disparities Report, information about care coordination from the 2005-2006 National Survey of Children With Special Health Care Needs[15] was presented. In this NHQR, we examine variation across States in receipt of coordinated care. For a child to qualify as receiving coordinated care, the parent had to report that they:

- Usually got as much help as wanted arranging or coordinating care.
- Were very satisfied with communication between the child's health care providers and his or her school, early intervention program, child care providers, or vocational education or rehabilitation program.
- Were very satisfied with the communication between the child's doctors and other health care providers.
- Overall, among children with special health care needs who required help with care coordination, 46.0% received the help they needed. Among States, the percentage receiving coordination ranged from 38.3% to 53.2%.
- The 13 States[LI] in the best quartile (highest rates of coordinated care) in 2005-2006 had a combined average rate of 50.5%. These States are primarily located in New England and the Midwest (Figure 5.7).

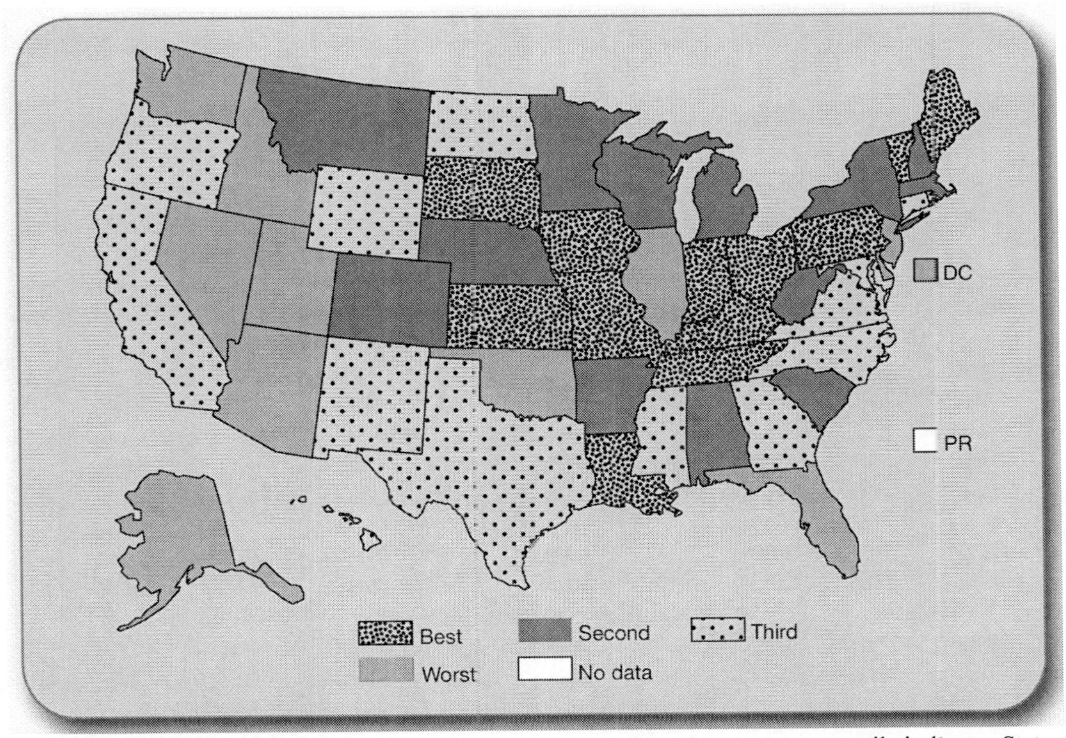

Key: Best quartile indicates States with highest rates of coordinated care; worst quartile indicates States with lowest rates.

Source: Health Resources and Services Administration, Maternal and Child Health Bureau; Centers for Disease Control and Prevention, National Center for Health Statistics, National Survey of Children With Special Health Care Needs, 2005-2006.]

Note: Analyses performed by the Child and Adolescent Health Measurement Initiative, Data Resource Center for Child and Adolescent Health (http://www.cshcndata.org).

Figure 5.7. State variation : Children with special health care needs who received coordinated care, 2005-2006

- Eleven States[LII] and the District of Columbia were in the worst quartile (lowest rates of coordinated care) in 2005-2006, with a combined average rate of 41.5%. These States are primarily located in the western United States.

REFERENCES

[1] Institute of Medicine. Envisioning the National Health Care Quality Report. *Washington, DC*: National Academy Press; 2001.

[2] Institute of Medicine. Crossing the quality chasm. a new health system for the 21st century. *Washington*, DC: National Academy Press; 2001.

[3] Stewart, M; Brown, JB; Donner A. et al. The impact of patient-centered care on outcomes. *J Fam Pract,* 2000 Sep, 49(9), 796-804.

[4] Anderson, EB. Patient-centeredness: a new approach. *Nephrol News Issues,* 2002 Nov, 16(12), 80-82.

[5] Little, P; Everitt, H; Williamson, I. et al. Observational study of effect of patient centredness and positive approach on outcomes of general practice consultations. *BMJ (Clinical research ed),* 2001 Oct 20, 323(7318), 908-11.

[6] Beck, RS; Daughtridge, R & Sloane, PD. Physician-patient communication in the primary care office: a systematic review. *J Am Board Fam Pract,* 2002 Jan-Feb, 15(1), 25-38.

[7] DiMatteo, MR. The role of the physician in the emerging health care environment. *West J Med*, 1998 May, 168(5), 328-33.

[8] Berry, LL; Seiders, K & Wilder, SS. Innovations in access to care: a patient-centered approach. *Ann Intern Med,* 2003 Oct 7, 139(7), 568-74.

[9] Bechel, DL; Myers, WA & Smith, DG. Does patient-centered care pay off? *Jt Comm J Qual Improv,* 2000 Jul, 26(7), 400-9.

[10] Shojania, K; McDonald, K; Wachter, R. et al. Closing the quality gap: a critical analysis of quality improvement strategies—Volume 7: care coordination. Rockville, MD: Agency for Healthcare Research and Quality; 2007. AHRQ Publication No. 04(07)-0051-7. Available at: http://www.ahrq.gov/clinic/tp/caregaptp.htm. Accessed on June 15, 2009.

[11] Davies, G; Williams, A & Larsen, K. et al. Coordinating primary health care: an analysis of the outcomes of a systematic review. *Med J Aust*, 2008 Apr 21;188(8):S65-S68.

[12] Quality insights. 2007 Patient Experiences in Primary Care. Massachusetts statewide results. Watertown: Massachusetts Health Quality Partners; 2009. Available at: http://www.mhqp.org/quality/pes/pesMASumm.asp?nav=031600.

[13] Agency for Healthcare Research and Quality. Healthcare Cost and Utilization Project. HCUPNet. 2006 national statistics outcomes for all discharges. Available at: http://www.hcupnet.ahrq.gov.

[14] McPherson, M; Arango, P & Fox, H. et al. A new definition of children with special health care needs. *Pediatrics,* 1998 Jul, 102(1 Pt 1), 137-40.

[15] Maternal and Child Health Bureau. The National Survey of Children With Special Health Care Needs, chartbook 2005-2006. Rockville, MD: Health Resources and Services Administration; 2008. Available at: http://mchb.hrsa.gov/cshcn05/index.htm. Accessed on August 12, 2009.

6. EFFICIENCY

Costs may not be on the minds of patients and providers when health care is being delivered. In fact, patients who have generous health insurance coverage rarely have to consider costs. But some patients are confronted with the costs of health care belatedly when they try to fill prescriptions that they discover they cannot afford or when expensive medical bills arrive. Medical bills contribute to many bankruptcies.[1] In addition, many Americans worry about not being able to afford health care. Quite a few report skipping care because of its cost.[2] People who buy their own health insurance, employers that provide health insurance coverage to their employees, and governments that fund health programs are made particularly aware of health care costs as they see these costs rising more quickly than wages, inflation, or economic growth.

One approach to containing the growth of health care costs is to improve the efficiency of the health care delivery system. This would allow finite health care resources to be used in a way that best supports high-quality care. Recent work examining variations in Medicare spending and quality shows that higher cost providers do not necessarily provide higher quality care, illustrating the potential for improvement.[3] It should be possible to maintain appropriate levels of health care provision without large increases in costs each year and to extract more value from each health care dollar. Improving efficiency in the Nation's health care system is an important component of the Department of Health and Human Services' (HHS) mission to support a better health care system. In support of this mission, this year's National Healthcare Quality Report (NHQR) continues to look at potential information sources and findings on efficiency in the U.S. health care system.

This year's NHQR outlines varying perspectives on efficiency and offers potential methods for measuring efficiency that respond to the NHQR's mandate to provide lawmakers in Congress with information on the performance of the U.S. health care system. This chapter does not attempt to provide a definitive framework for efficiency; nor does it provide an exhaustive list of potential measures of efficiency. Rather, the Agency for Healthcare Research and Quality (AHRQ) hopes that this chapter will stimulate productive dialog on health care efficiency. AHRQ intends this chapter to be part of an evolving national discussion on measuring efficiency in the U.S. health care system that will be reviewed, revised, and presented in future reports.

Measures

Part of the discussion about how to improve efficiency involves the question about how best to measure it. Varying perspectives and definitions of health care efficiency exist, and the lack of consensus on what constitutes appropriate measurement of efficiency has stymied efforts to report on this area.

To improve understanding of efficiency measures, AHRQ commissioned the RAND Corporation to systematically review measures of efficiency and to assess their potential to be tracked and reported at various levels.[4] The RAND report provides a typology of efficiency measures that emphasizes the multiple perspectives on efficiency. It also points out that measures must be considered from the standpoint of what the measuring organization is and what its goal is in assessing efficiency.

In considering efficiency measures, AHRQ also built on another report that examined the question of efficiency from the cost-of-waste point of view. In that report, the authors outline another common typology for efficiency measurement: the tracking of overuse, underuse, and misuse in the health care system.[5]

This chapter presents measures from the population and provider perspective to provide some insight into health care efficiency. They are:

- Trends in potentially avoidable hospitalizations and costs (population perspective).
- Disparities in potentially avoidable hospitalizations (population perspective).
- Potentially avoidable hospitalizations among Medicare home health and nursing home patients (population perspective).
- Potentially avoidable hospitalizations and emergency department encounters for congestive heart failure (CHF) (population perspective).
- Rehospitalization for CHF for selected States (population perspective).
- Reduction of unnecessary costs (population perspective).
- Trends in hospital efficiency (provider perspective).

Consensus has yet to emerge about the appropriate framework and acceptable measures of efficiency, and the examples provided are designed to stimulate productive ongoing discussion about health care efficiency. We anticipate reporting the trends in potentially avoidable hospitalizations and costs and trends in hospital efficiency measures in future NHQRs. We also plan to include periodic focuses on particular conditions. However, some of the estimates that we are making available in this year's chapter will only appear intermittently in the future.

Findings

Trends in Potentially Avoidable Hospitalizations and Costs

To address potentially avoidable hospitalizations and costs from the population perspective, data on ambulatory care-sensitive conditions are summarized here using the AHRQ Prevention Quality Indicators (PQIs). Not all hospitalizations that the AHRQ PQIs track are preventable, but ambulatory care-sensitive conditions are those for which good outpatient care can prevent the need for hospitalization or for which early intervention can prevent complications or more severe disease. The AHRQ PQIs track these conditions using hospital discharge data. Hospitalizations for acute conditions, such as dehydration or pneumonia, are distinguished from hospitalizations for chronic conditions, such as diabetes or CHF.

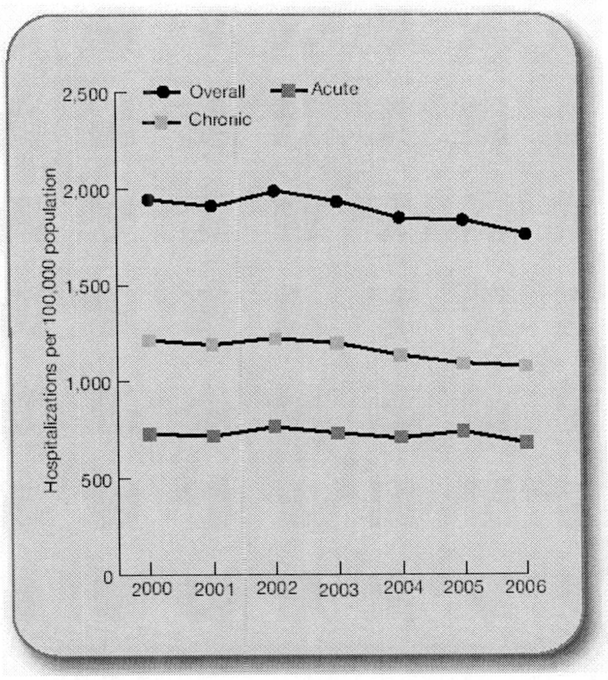

Source: Agency for Healthcare Research and Quality, Healthcare Cost and Utilization Project, Nationwide Inpatient Sample, 2000-2006.

Note: Data are for adults age 18 and over. Annual rates are adjusted for age and gender.

Figure 6.1. National trends in potentially avoidable hospitalization rates for adults, by type of hospitalization, 2000-2006

For this analysis, total hospital charges were converted to costs using Healthcare Cost and Utilization Project (HCUP) cost-to-charge ratios based on hospital accounting reports from the Centers for Medicare & Medicaid Services. Therefore, cost estimates in this section refer to hospital costs for providing care, but do not include either payers' costs or costs for physician care that are billed separately.

- From 2000 to 2006, overall rates of avoidable hospitalizations decreased significantly, from 1,944 per 100,000 to 1,761 per 100,000 (Figure 6.1).
- This decline is largely attributable to avoidable hospitalizations for chronic conditions, which decreased significantly, from 1,213 per 100,000 to 1,078 per 100,000.
- Avoidable hospitalizations for acute conditions did not change significantly from 2000 to 2006.
- From 2000 to 2003, total national hospital costs associated with potentially avoidable hospitalizations adjusted for inflation[LIII] increased from $27.9 billion to $31.9 billion (Figure 6.2). Costs then declined to $30.1 billion in 2006.
- These changes are largely attributable to avoidable hospitalizations for chronic conditions, with national hospital costs that increased from $17.6 billion to $20.3 billion between 2000 and 2003 and then declined to $19.2 billion in 2006.

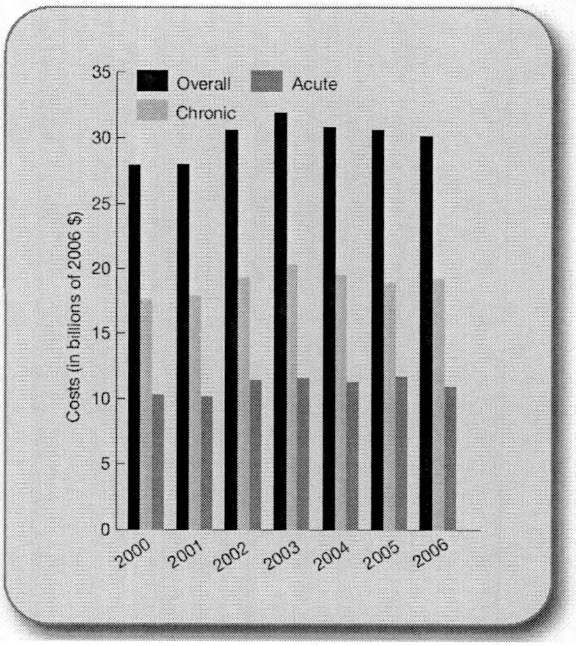

Source: Agency for Healthcare Research and Quality, Healthcare Cost and Utilization Project, Nationwide Inpatient Sample, 2000-2006.

Note: Data are for adults age 18 and over. Annual rates are adjusted for age and gender. Costs are adjusted for inflation.

Figure 6.2. Total national costs associated with potentially avoidable hospitalizations, 2000-2006

- National hospital costs for avoidable hospitalizations for acute conditions did not change significantly from 2000 to 2006.

Disparities in Potentially Avoidable Hospitalizations

Relatively little work has focused on the use of efficiency measures to assess disparities in the delivery of health care. In considering efficiency measures for the NHQR and the National Healthcare Disparities Report (NHDR), we assessed their ability to support analyses by race, ethnicity, and socioeconomic status (SES). Most measures did not allow assessment of disparities, so we have not included a section on efficiency in the NHDR. However, data for one efficiency measure, potentially avoidable hospitalizations, were deemed to be of sufficient quality to assess disparities.

A critical caveat should be noted. Comparatively high rates of potentially avoidable hospitalizations may reflect inefficiency in the health care system. Therefore, groups of patients should not be "blamed" for receiving less efficient care. Instead, examining disparities in efficiency may help make the business case for addressing disparities in care. Investments that reduce disparities in access to high-quality outpatient care may help reduce rates of avoidable hospitalizations among groups that have high rates.

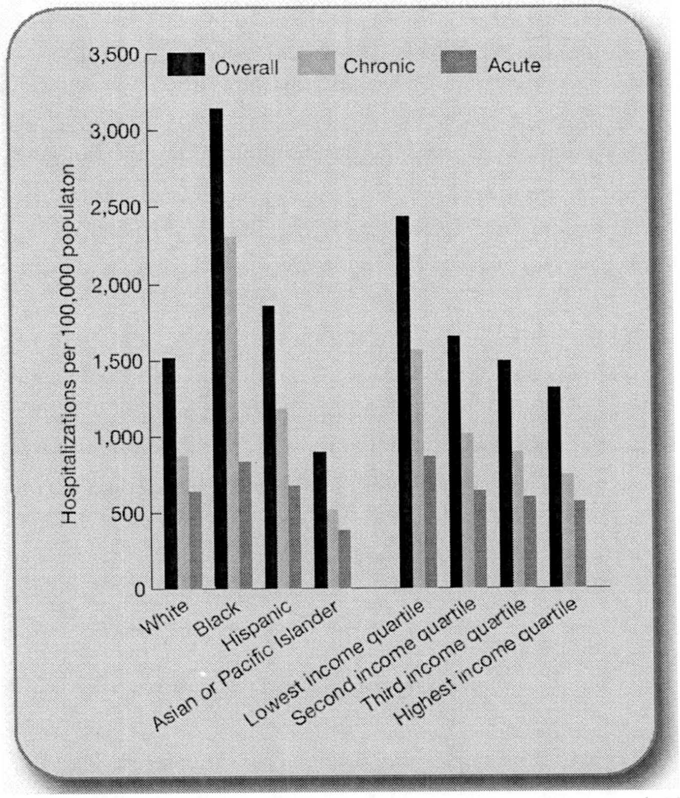

Source: Agency for Healthcare Research and Quality, Healthcare Cost and Utilization Project, Nationwide Inpatient Sample, 2006.

Note: Data are for adults age 18 and over. Annual rates are adjusted for age and gender. White, Black, and Asian or Pacific Islander are non-Hispanic. Income quartiles based on median income of Zip Code of patient's residence.

Figure 6.3. Potentially avoidable hospitalization rates for adults, by race/ethnicity and area income, 2006

- Rates of avoidable hospitalizations overall and avoidable hospitalizations for chronic conditions were higher among Blacks and Hispanics compared with Whites. Rates were lower among Asians and Pacific Islanders (APIs) compared with Whites (Figure 6.3).
- Rates of avoidable hospitalizations overall and avoidable hospitalizations for chronic conditions were higher among residents of areas in the lowest, second, and third income quartiles compared with residents of areas in the highest income quartile.
- Rates of avoidable hospitalizations for acute conditions were higher among Blacks compared with Whites and among residents of areas in the lowest and second income quartiles compared with residents of areas in the highest income quartile.

Potentially Avoidable Hospitalizations among Medicare Home Health and Nursing Home Patients

Many patients are hospitalized while receiving care from home health agencies and nursing homes, with resulting high costs and care transition problems. A number of these hospitalizations of nursing home and home health patients are appropriate. However, some hospital admissions could be prevented with better primary care and monitoring in these settings, or the patient could receive appropriate treatment in a less resource-intense setting.

Using the AHRQ Prevention Quality Indicators (PQIs), we track potentially avoidable hospitalizations among Medicare patients occurring within 30 days of the start of home health or nursing home care. These patients may differ from patients discussed earlier in this chapter who are predominantly admitted for avoidable conditions from home. At home, some are receiving appropriate primary care and others have not visited a health care provider for years.

In contrast, Medicare home health and nursing home patients have regular contact with health providers, which should reduce rates of avoidable hospitalization. However, these patients are also more acutely ill, may become seriously ill when affected by a new illness, and may have multiple comorbidities. Medicare patients in these settings often have been hospitalized recently. Therefore, an avoidable hospitalization may represent a return to the hospital, perhaps against the expectation that the patient was no longer in need of acute care.

For application to home health and nursing home settings, the potentially avoidable stays are identified within a defined time period, 30 days, from the home health or nursing home admission date. If a patient is hospitalized more than once in that period, only the first stay is recognized for the measure.

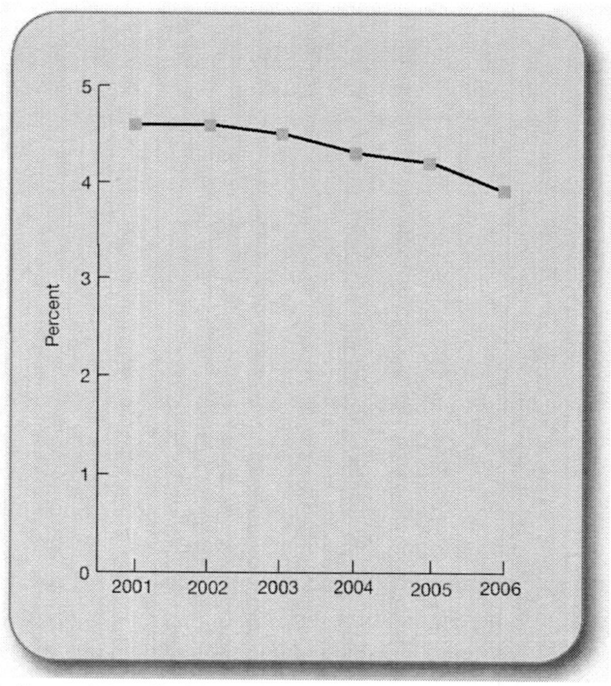

Source: Centers for Medicare & Medicaid Services, Outcome and Assessment Information Set linked with Medicare Part A claims (100%), 2001-2006.

Denominator: Adult nonmaternity patients starting an episode of skilled home health care.

Note: Rates standardized to the 2006 patient population according to Medicare enrollment category.

Figure 6.4. Medicare home health patients with potentially avoidable hospitalizations within 30 days of start of care, 2001-2006

Data on home health patients come from Medicare fee-for-service (FFS) home health claims and Outcome and Assessment Information Set (OASIS) patient assessment information. Data on nursing home patients come from Medicare skilled nursing facility (SNF) FFS claims and Minimum Data Set (MDS) patient assessment information. These data are linked with Medicare Part A acute care hospital claims to determine hospitalizations for potentially avoidable conditions.

- Between 2001 and 2006, hospitalizations within 30 days of home health episode start for potentially avoidable conditions declined from 4.6% to 3.9%.
- Between 2000 and 2005, hospitalizations within 30 days of nursing home admission for potentially avoidable conditions increased for short-stay nursing home residents but declined slightly for long-stay nursing home residents.

Potentially Avoidable Hospitalizations and Emergency Department Encounters for Congestive Heart Failure

Potentially preventable, high-cost encounters with the medical system occur not only in hospitals, but also in emergency departments (EDs). There were more than 120 million ED encounters in 2006. ED crowding, boarding (i.e., holding patients until an inpatient bed is available), and ambulance diversion have become more prevalent and have given rise to increasing concerns about the quality of care delivered in EDs.

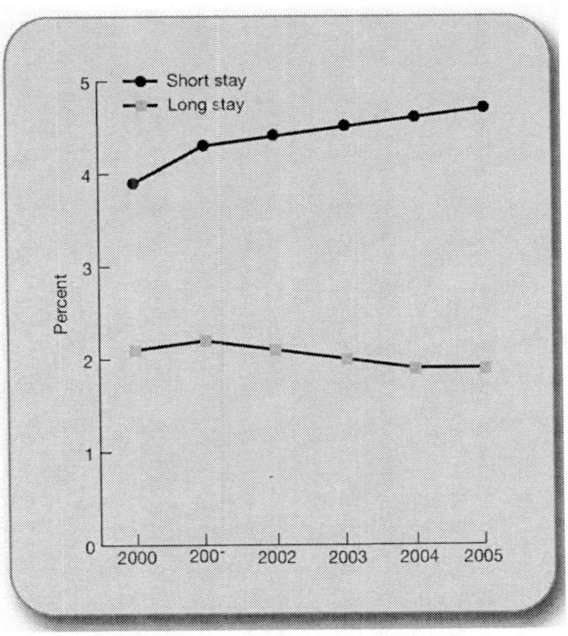

Source: Centers for Medicare & Medicaid Services, Minimum Data Set, 2000-2005 linked with Medicare Part A claims (100%).

Denominator: Short-stay residents are those who met the Medicare skilled nursing facility (SNF) criteria for nursing home admission; long-stay residents are nursing home admissions that did not meet Medicare SNF criteria.

Figure 6.5. Short-stay and long-stay nursing home residents with potentially avoidable hospitalizations within 30 days of admission, 2000-2005

Congestive heart failure (CHF) is an ambulatory care-sensitive condition. Patients typically need to restrict their intake of salt, take their medications regularly, and monitor their weight. Good primary care can help patients with self-management and make adjustments to treatment before exacerbations in CHF become severe and require emergent attention.

Some hospitalizations and ED encounters cannot be avoided, but appropriate ambulatory care can help keep some patients from having to visit an ED or from being hospitalized. Reducing potentially avoidable ED encounters, in particular, holds promise for reducing cost, improving quality, and enhancing efficiency. For this analysis, the CHF measure from the the AHRQ PQI software was applied to the 2005 HCUP Nationwide Inpatient Sample (NIS) and the Nationwide Emergency Department Sample (NEDS).

- The South had a rate of inpatient stays for CHF that was significantly higher than the rate for the Northeast. The West had a lower rate. The rate for the Midwest was statistically indistinguishable from the rate for the Northeast (Figure 6.6).
- The South had a rate of ED visits for CHF that was significantly higher than the rate for the Northeast. The rates for the Midwest and the West were statistically indistinguishable from the rate for the Northeast.

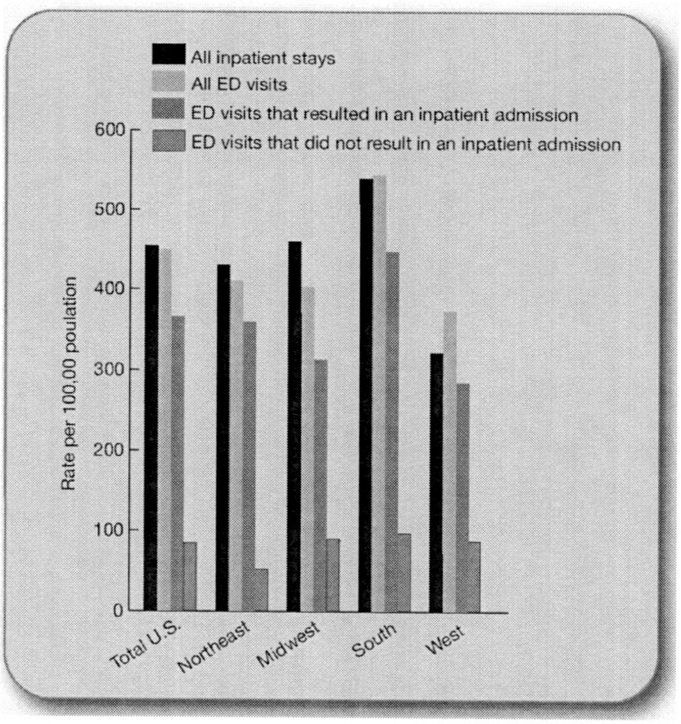

Key: ED = emergency department.

Source: Agency for Healthcare Research and Quality, Healthcare Cost and Utilization Project, Nationwide Inpatient Sample and Nationwide Emergency Department Sample, 2005.

Note: Data are for adults age 18 and over. Annual rates are adjusted for age and gender.

Figure 6.6. Potentially avoidable hospitalizations and emergency department encounters for congestive heart failure, national and regional estimates, 2005

- The South had a rate of ED visits that resulted in an inpatient admission for CHF that was significantly higher than the rate for the Northeast. The West had a lower rate. The rate for the Midwest was statistically indistinguishable from the rate for the Northeast.
- The South, West, and Midwest had rates of ED visits that did not result in an inpatient admission for CHF that were significantly higher than the rate for the Northeast.

Table 6.1. Rehospitalizations for Congestive Heart Failure, 14 States, 2006

Age category	State	Hospitalized CHF patients with rehospitalization for CHF	Average cost of rehospitalization
Ages 18-64	State A	3.6%	DSU
	State B	6.1%	$11,030
	State C	8.3%	$8,753
	State D	8.3%	$9,925
	State E	8.5%	$12,424
	State F	8.6%	$10,809
	State G	9.1%	$10,865
	State H	9.9%	$10,055
	State I	9.9%	$11,049
	State J	10.1%	$9,583
	State K	11.4%	$9,488
	State L	11.5%	$8,599
	State M	11.7%	$12,908
	State N	11.8%	$8,058
Age 65+	State A	4.4%	$8,907
	State D	6.8%	$9,867
	State I	6.9%	$9,800
	State C	8.4%	$8,139
	State E	8.8%	$7,901
	State B	8.8%	$9,633
	State J	9.3%	$9,390
	State N	9.4%	$7,631
	State F	9.4%	$9,926
	State M	9.5%	$12,692
	State K	9.8%	$9,047
	State H	10.0%	$8,821
	State L	10.0%	$7,351
	State G	10.6%	$8,891

Key: DSU = data statistically unreliable.

Source: Agency for Healthcare Research and Quality, Healthcare Cost and Utilization Project, State Inpatient Databases, 2006.

Note: Data are for adults age 18 and over. The data for State A were insufficient for determining the average cost of rehospitalization.

Rehospitalization for Congestive Heart Failure

To gain further insight into the population perspective of potentially avoidable hospitalizations and costs, data on rehospitalization rates for CHF for 14 States in 2006 are summarized here. Rehospitalization for CHF signals a worsened state of illness for patients and is more resource intensive than outpatient treatment. Although some rehospitalizations for CHF cannot be prevented, CHF is a condition for which good outpatient care and early intervention can help prevent rehospitalization.

The estimates below are derived from data for 14 States participating in the HCUP State Inpatient Databases. They are based on all CHF admissions from January 1 to November 30, 2006. Rehospitalizations are defined as admissions to any hospital in that State with a principal diagnosis of CHF within 30 days of the discharge date of an index CHF admission. For this analysis, total hospital charges were converted to costs using HCUP cost-to-charge ratios based on hospital accounting reports from the Centers for Medicare & Medicaid Services. Therefore, cost estimates in this section refer to hospital costs.

- The percentage of State-level CHF hospitalizations resulting in rehospitalization for CHF ranged from a low of 3.6% to a high of 11.8% for patients ages 18-64 and from a low of 4.4% to a high of 10.6% for patients age 65 and over. State A had the lowest percentage for both age groups (Table 6.1).
- Costs for a rehospitalization for CHF where the index hospitalization was for CHF ranged from a low of $8,058 to a high of $12,908 for patients ages 18-64 and from a low of $7,351 to a high of $12,692 for patients age 65 and over.
- Costs for a rehospitalization for CHF where the index hospitalization was for CHF were generally lower in the Medicare-eligible population than in those ages 18-64.

It is important to note that the figures reported above are not national estimates and that no conclusions about national trends should be inferred. The States in the analysis account for about 32% of all adult discharges for CHF in the Nation and provide an indication of the general trend that readmissions for CHF may be following.

Reduction of Unnecessary Costs

This section of the chapter highlights waste and opportunities to reduce unnecessary costs. Waste can include overuse, underuse, or misuse of health care services. An example of overuse is prostate-specific antigen (PSA) screening among men age 75 and over, which the U.S. Preventive Services Task Force (USPSTF) recently recommended against.[6] Our analyses of the 2005 National Health Interview Survey indicate that there were approximately 1.7 million men age 75 and over with no history of prostate cancer who reported having a routine PSA test in the past year. This makes up 42.8% of all men age 75 and over.

There is concern that administration of the PSA test in men age 75 and over will lead to false positives and subsequent unnecessary treatments. Reductions in costs and improvements in quality should result from reductions in unnecessary PSA screening. Patient and provider education is regarded as the key to reducing the overutilization of PSA screening.

Another overused treatment that can be reduced through education is the use of antibiotics to treat the common cold. Taking antibiotics does not treat or relieve symptoms of the common cold and may lead to the development of antibiotic-resistant bacterial infections.

Although antibiotic prescribing patterns are slowly improving, inappropriate use of antibiotics for the common cold is still a concern.[7] Children have the highest rates of antibiotic use and the highest rates of bacterial infection with antibiotic-resistant bacterial pathogens.[8]

- In 2006-2007, the overall rate of antibiotics prescribed at visits with a diagnosis of the common cold stood at 59.9 per 10,000 population, which is below the Healthy People 2010 target of reducing rates to no more than 126.8 per 10,000 (Figure 6.7).
- From 1998-1999 to 2006-2007, the rate of antibiotic prescription at visits with a diagnosis of common cold decreased overall and for people of all age groups.
- In 2006-2007, all age groups were below the Healthy People 2010 target.

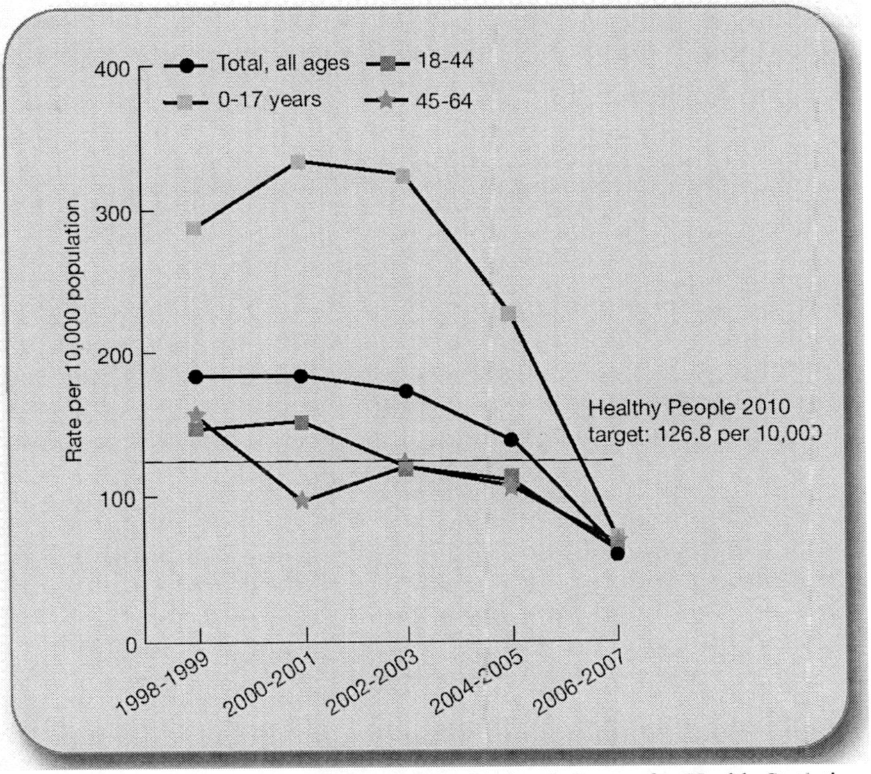

Source: Centers for Disease Control and Prevention, National Center for Health Statistics, National Ambulatory Medical Care Survey and National Hospital Ambulatory Medical Care Survey, 1998-2007.

Denominator: U.S. noninstitutionalized population.

Figure 6.7. Visits with antibiotics prescribed for a diagnosis of common cold per 10,000 population, 1998-2007.

Trends in Hospital Efficiency

Significant attention has been paid to cost variations across providers and across the country. Yet it is often difficult to separate out costs that reflect differences among providers in outputs, patient burden of illness,[LIV] or care quality. To address the provider perspective, hospital cost efficiency is examined using a technique from the field of econometrics that can account for such differences.[LV] This analysis uses data from the American Hospital Association Annual Survey and from Medicare Cost Reports, as well as data derived from the application of AHRQ Quality Indicators software to HCUP data and the application of comorbidity software to HCUP data.

Here, hospital efficiency is defined as the ratio of best practice costs to total observed costs. For example, given the types and quantities of outputs a hospital produces, the input prices it pays, its case mix, its quality, and its market characteristics, a theoretical best practice hospital might incur expenses amounting to $90 million. A comparison hospital in an identical situation with total expenses of $100 million would have an estimated cost efficiency of 90%.

Cost-efficiency estimates have been converted to index numbers with a base of 100 for the year 2002 as a way to place less emphasis on the specific magnitude of estimated hospital efficiency than on its general trend.

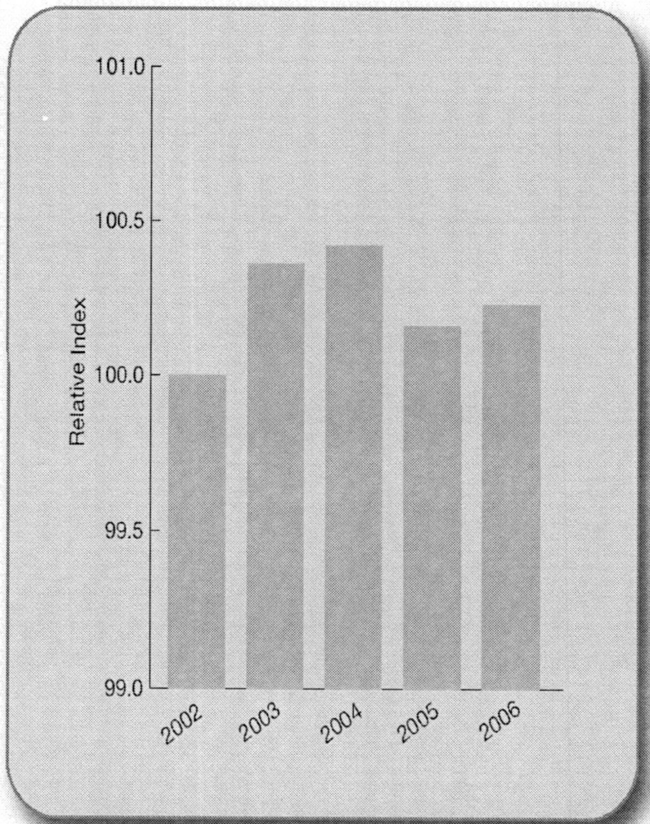

Source: Agency for Healthcare Research and Quality. Analysis based on 1,382 urban general community hospitals with data in the Healthcare Cost and Utilization Project, State Inpatient Databases. Refer to Chapter 1, Introduction and Methods, for further details.

Figure 6.8. Average estimated relative hospital cost-efficiency index for a selected sample of urban general community hospitals, 2002-2006

Table 6.2. Correlates of Hospital Cost Efficiency

Measure	Estimate	Standard deviation
Cost per case mix-adjusted admission:		
Top quartile of hospital cost efficiency	$4,740	$1,321
Bottom quartile of hospital cost efficiency	$6,581	$2,612
Full-time equivalent employees per case mix-adjusted admission:		
Top quartile of hospital cost efficiency	.042	0.01
Bottom quartile of hospital cost efficiency	.053	0.02
Average length of stay (days):		
Top quartile of hospital cost efficiency	5.08	1.47
Bottom quartile of hospital cost efficiency	5.14	1.79
Operating margin:		
Top quartile of hospital cost efficiency	.008	0.12
Bottom quartile of hospital cost efficiency	-.072	0.23

Source: American Hospital Association Annual Survey of Hospitals and Medicare Cost Reports, 2002-2006.

- Estimated urban hospital cost efficiency increased slightly from 2002 to 2004 but decreased slightly in 2005 for a selected sample of urban general community hospitals. It increased again in 2006 (Figure 6.8).
- The most cost-efficient hospitals (i.e., hospitals in the highest quartile of estimated cost efficiency) compared favorably with the least cost-efficient hospitals (i.e., hospitals in the lowest quartile of estimated cost efficiency) on a number of important variables. The most cost-efficient hospitals had lower costs and fewer full-time-equivalent employees per case mix-adjusted admission compared with the least cost-efficient hospitals. The most cost-efficient hospitals also had a shorter average length of stay, although the difference was not statistically significant (Table 6.2).
- The most cost-efficient hospitals had a higher operating margin than the least cost-efficient hospitals (Table 6.2).

It is important to note that the figures reported above are not national estimates and that no conclusions about national trends should be inferred. However, the hospitals in the analysis represent about 55% of all nonFederal urban general community hospitals and therefore provide an indication of the general trend that cost efficiency may be following.

REFERENCES

[1] Himmelstein, DU; Thorne, D; Warren, E. et al. Medical bankruptcy in the United States, 2007: results of a national study. *Am J Med,* 2009 Aug, 122(8), 741-6.

[2] Kaiser health tracking poll. Washington, DC: The Henry J. Kaiser Family Foundation; February 2009. Available at: http://www.kff.org/kaiserpolls/upload/7866.pdf. Accessed on August 12, 2009.

[3] Fisher, ES; Wennberg, DE & Stukel, TA. et al. The implications of regional variations in Medicare spending. Part 1: the content, quality, and accessibility of care. *Ann Intern Med,* 2003 Feb 18, 138(4), 273-87.
[4] McGlynn, EA. Identifying, categorizing, and evaluating health care efficiency measures: . Rockville, MD: Agency for Healthcare Research and Quality; 2008. AHRQ Publication No. 08-0030. Available at: http://www.ahrq.gov/qual/efficiency. Accessed on December 8, 2009.
[5] James, B; Bayley, KB. Cost of poor quality or waste in integrated delivery system settings (Final report prepared under Contract No. 290-00-0018-11). Rockville, MD: Agency for Healthcare Research and Quality; 2006. Available at: www.ahrq.gov/RESEARCH/costpoorids.pdf. Accessed on August 13, 2009.
[6] Screening for prostate cancer. Rockville, MD: Agency for Healthcare Research and Quality; 2008. Available at: http://www.ahrq.gov/CLINIC/uspstf/uspsprca.htm. Accessed on August 13, 2009.
[7] Nash, DR; Harman, J; Wald, ER. et al. Antibiotic prescribing by primary care physicians for children with upper respiratory tract infections. *Arch Pediatr Adolesc Med,* 2002 Nov, 156(11), 1114-9.
[8] Perz, JF; Craig, AS; Coffey, CS. et al. Changes in antibiotic prescribing for children after a community-wide campaign. *JAMA,* 2002 Jun 19, 287(23), 3103-9.
[9] Elixhauser, A; Steiner, C; Harris, R. et al. Comorbidity measures for use with administratiove data. *Med Care,* 1998, 36, 8-27.
[10] Mutter, R; Rosko, M; Wang, H. Measuring hospital inefficiency: the effects of controlling for quality and patient burden of illness. *Health Serv Res,* 2008, 43, 1992-2013.

End Notes

[I] The HHS Interagency Work Group, which represents 18 HHS agencies and offices, provides advice and support to AHRQ and the National Reports Team.

[II] Because of this high level of performance, these measures cannot improve further to a significant degree. To prevent this ceiling effect from distorting calculations of rate of change over time, these measures were retired from the measure set tracked in this chapter.

[III] Some data sources do not distinguish "self-pay" patients with no insurance from patients who have insurance but pay for services out of pocket, either because a service is not covered or they choose to pay.

[IV] NHQR data can be accessed through NHQRDRnet, an online tool that provides Internet users with an opportunity to specify dimensions of analysis and produce data tables. NHQRDRnet is available through the AHRQ Web site at http://nhqrnet.ahrq.gov.

[V] Go to Chapter 1, Introduction and Methods, in the 2006 NHQR for more detailed information about these and other methods used to calculate composite measures used in the reports.

[VI] The vaccines included in this measure are based on the corresponding Healthy People 2010 objective and do not include all vaccines currently recommended for children. Specifically, varicella vaccine and vaccines added after 1998 to the recommended schedule for children up to 35 months of age are not included in this composite measure.

[VII] $[(Pn/Po)^{1/N}-1]x100$ where Pn=variable at later time period, Po=variable at earlier time period, and N=number of years in interval. From the entry for Average Annual Rate of Change in Appendix II, Definitions and Methods, *Health, United States, 2008*. Available at: http://www.cdc.gov/nchs/hus.htm.

[VIII] More precisely, to calculate annual rate of change, the natural log of each year's data point is entered into a linear regression model.

[IX] Throughout this chapter, total cost equals cost of medical care (direct cost) and economic costs of morbidity and mortality (indirect cost). Direct costs are defined as "personal health care expenditures for hospital and nursing home care, drugs, home care, and physician and other professional services."[4]

[X] Cost-effectiveness is measured here by the average net cost of each quality-adjusted life year (QALY) that is saved by the provision of a particular health intervention. QALYs are a measure of survival adjusted for its value: 1 year in perfect health is equal to 1.0 QALY, while a year in poor health would be something less than 1.0. A lower cost per QALY saved indicates a greater degree of cost-effectiveness.

[XI] Medicare does not cover all health care costs. Medicare beneficiaries can purchase supplemental insurance from private insurance companies to help pay for coinsurance, copayments, deductibles, and noncovered services. Low-income beneficiaries may receive assistance from Medicaid and other public insurance programs to help pay for costs not covered by Medicare. Beneficiaries with Medicare typically pay out of pocket for costs related to premiums, deductibles, coinsurance, copayments, and noncovered services.

[XII] The States are Connecticut, Delaware, Maine, Maryland, Massachusetts, Michigan, Minnesota, New Hampshire, New York, Rhode Island, Tennessee, and Vermont.

[XIII] The States are Arkansas, Idaho, Indiana, Mississippi, Missouri, Montana, Nevada, New Mexico, Oklahoma, Texas, Utah, and Wyoming.

[XIV] HbA1c, or glycosylated hemoglobin, is a measure of average levels of glucose in the blood.

[XV] The States are Alaska, California, Florida, Louisiana, Mississippi, Nevada, New Mexico, Ohio, Oklahoma, South Carolina, and Texas. Data on this measure were not available for Connecticut, District of Columbia, Illinois, Kansas, Maryland, Massachusetts, Nebraska, Puerto Rico, Rhode Island, and Wisconsin.

[XVI] The States are Arkansas, Georgia, Kentucky, Nevada, North Carolina, Ohio, Oklahoma, South Carolina, Tennessee, and West Virginia. Data on this measure were not available for Alabama, Alaska, Delaware, District of Columbia, Idaho, Louisiana, Mississippi, Montana, New Mexico, North Dakota, Pennsylvania, Puerto Rico, and Wyoming.

[XVII] The States are Nevada, Ohio, Oklahoma, and South Carolina.

[XVIII] Blood pressure control guidelines were updated in 2005. Previously, having a blood pressure reading of <140/90 mm Hg was considered under control. For this measure, the new threshold of <140/80 mm Hg has been applied to historic data for the sake of consistency and comparability.

[XIX] The States are California, Colorado, Massachusetts, Michigan, Minnesota, New Hampshire, New Jersey, North Dakota, Pennsylvania, South Dakota, Vermont, Wisconsin, and Wyoming.

[XX] The States are Connecticut, Florida, Georgia, Kentucky, Louisiana, Mississippi, New Mexico, North Carolina, Oklahoma, Oregon, and South Carolina.

[XXI] The States are Florida, Georgia, Kansas, Kentucky, Louisiana, Maine, Massachusetts, Mississippi, New Mexico, Pennsylvania, Tennessee, and Utah.

[XXII] The States are Arkansas, Hawaii, Iowa, Kansas, Nebraska, Nevada, Oklahoma, Utah, and Vermont. Data on this measure were not available for Alabama, Alaska, Delaware, District of Columbia, Idaho, Indiana, Louisiana, Mississippi, Montana, New Mexico, North Dakota, Ohio, Pennsylvania, South Dakota, and Wyoming.

[XXIII] The States are Kansas and Utah.

[XIV] Includes costs of domestic care, housing and other financial assistance, prevention, and research.

[XXV] The States are Colorado, Kansas, Michigan, Minnesota, Nebraska, Oregon, Utah, Washington, West Virginia, and Wisconsin.

[XXVI] The States are Delaware, Florida, Georgia, Louisiana, Maryland, Mississippi, New Jersey, New York, and South Carolina.

[XXVII] In this chapter, children are defined as individuals under age 18.

[XXVIII] The childhood immunization series includes vaccinations for diphtheria-tetanus-pertussis, measles-mumps-rubella, inactivated polio virus, *Haemophilus influenzae* type B, hepatitis B, and varicella. "Cost saving" indicates that childhood immunizations are one of very few services that save more money than they cost.

[XXIX] Compared with other common preventive services such as screening for breast cancer or hypertension, screening for problem drinking is highly cost-effective.

[XXX] The States are California, Connecticut, Delaware, Georgia, Hawaii, Illinois, Maryland, Massachusetts, New Jersey, New York, Rhode Island, and Texas.

[XXXI] The States are Alaska, Arizona, Colorado, Idaho, Kentucky, Montana, Nevada, New Mexico, Oklahoma, Oregon, South Dakota, Utah, and Wyoming.

[XXXII] Chronic lower respiratory diseases include emphysema and chronic bronchitis.

[XXXIII] The States are Idaho, Iowa, Maine, Montana, Nebraska, New Hampshire, New Jersey, Oklahoma, South Carolina, South Dakota, Vermont, Wisconsin, and Wyoming.

[XXXIV] The States are Alaska, Arizona, Georgia, Hawaii, Kansas, Louisiana, Maryland, Mississippi, Nevada, New Mexico, and Washington.

[XXXV] ADLs consist of basic self-care tasks, such as bathing, dressing, eating, transferring, using the toilet, and walking.

[XXXVI] IADLs consist of tasks needed for a person to live independently, such as shopping, doing housework, preparing meals, taking medications, using the telephone, and managing money.

XXXVII The States are Georgia, Kentucky, Maine, Maryland, Mississippi, Nevada, New Jersey, Rhode Island, South Carolina, Tennessee, Utah, Virginia, and West Virginia.

XXXVIII The States are Alaska, Arizona, Delaware, Iowa, Minnesota, New York, Oregon, Texas, and Wyoming.

XXXIX Medicare FFS patients represent only a portion of all home health patients.

XL Cost estimates for nursing home and home health services include only costs for freestanding skilled nursing facilities, nursing homes, and home health agencies and not those that are hospital based.

XLI The States are Alaska, Delaware, Iowa, Kansas, Maine, Nebraska, New Hampshire, North Dakota, Rhode Island, Virginia, and Wisconsin.

XLII The States are Arkansas, California, Colorado, Florida, Kentucky, Louisiana, Mississippi, New Mexico, Ohio, Oklahoma, South Carolina, Tennessee, and Utah.

XLIII "Short stay" refers to residents who are admitted to a facility and stay fewer than 30 days; these admissions, also referred to as "postacute," typically follow an acute care hospitalization.

XLIV "Long stay" or "chronic care" refers to residents who enter a nursing facility typically because they are no longer able to care for themselves at home; they tend to remain in the facility from several months to several years. High-risk residents are those who are in a coma, do not get the nutrients they need to maintain good skin health, or cannot change position on their own. Low-risk residents are active, can change positions, and are getting the nutrients they need to maintain good skin health.

XLV This survey provides unique insight into end-of-life care and captures information about a large percentage of hospice patients but is limited by nonrandom data collection and a response rate of about 40%. Survey questions were answered by family members, who might not be fully aware of the patients' wishes and concerns. These limitations should be considered when interpreting these findings.

XLVI This measure is based on responses from patients' family members, who may or may not be able to determine whether the right amount of medicine for pain was administered.

XLVII The States are Delaware, Maine, Massachusetts, Michigan, Montana, Nebraska, New Hampshire, New Jersey, North Carolina, South Carolina, South Dakota, Vermont, and Wisconsin.

XLVIII The States are Arizona, California, Georgia, Idaho, Louisiana, Mississippi, Nevada, New Mexico, Oregon, Texas, and Utah.

XLIX Drugs that should always be avoided for older patients include barbiturates, flurazepam, meprobamate, chlorpropamide, meperidine, pentazocine, trimethobenzamide, belladonna alkaloids, dicyclomine, hyoscyamine, and propantheline. Drugs that should often or always be avoided for older patients include carisoprodol, chlorzoxazone, cyclobenzaprine, metaxalone, methocarbamol, amitriptyline, chlordiazepoxide, diazepam, doxepin, indomethacin, dipyridamole, ticlopidine, methyldopa, reserpine, disopyramide, oxybutynin, chlorpheniramine, cyproheptadine, diphenhydramine, hydroxyzine, promethazine, and propoxyphene.

L For example, Title VI of the Civil Rights Act of 1964, 42 U.S.C. 2000d, may require the practitioner or hospital to provide language interpreters and translate vital documents for limited-English-proficient people. Section 504 of the Rehabilitation Act of 1973, 29 U.S.C. 794, may require sign language interpreters, materials in Braille, or accessible electronic formats for people with disabilities.

LI The States are Indiana, Iowa, Kansas, Kentucky, Louisiana, Maine, Missouri, Ohio, Pennsylvania, Rhode Island, South Dakota, Tennessee, and Vermont.

LII The States are Alaska, Arizona, Delaware, Florida, Idaho, Illinois, Nevada, New Jersey, Oklahoma, Utah, and Washington.

LIII The inflation adjustment was done using the gross domestic product implicit price deflator.

LIV This analysis controls for the following components that Elixhauser, et al. (1998) contend are part of patient burden of illness: (1) primary reason for admission to the hospital, (2) severity of the principal diagnosis, (3) iatrogenic complications, and (4) comorbidities that are unrelated to the primary diagnosis but have a substantial impact on both the resources used to treat the patient and the outcomes of the care provided.[9]

LV Stochastic frontier analysis (SFA) is the technique used in this analysis. SFA can estimate best practice costs as the value total costs would be if full efficiency were attained. The hospital-level "cost efficiency" estimates that SFA produces measure whether output is obtained using the fewest inputs (i.e., technical efficiency), as well as whether output is produced using the optimal mix of inputs, given prices (i.e., allocative efficiency), the size of a hospital's operations (i.e., scale efficiency), and the range of a hospital's operations (i.e., scope efficiency), including possible overspecialization or overdiversification.[10]

INDEX

A

B

C

D

E

F

G

H

I

K

L

M

N

O

P

Q

R

S